The Heart of Health

The Heart of Health

Embracing Life with Your Mind and Spirit

Mary I. Farr

John Wiley & Sons, Inc.

New York • Chichester • Weinheim • Brisbane • Singapore • Toronto

Published by John Wiley & Sons, Inc.
Published simultaneously in Canada

The information contained in this book is not intended to serve as a replacement for professional medical advice. Any use of the information in this book is at the reader's discretion. The author and the publisher specifically disclaim any and all liability arising directly or indirectly from the use or application of any information contained in this book. A health care professional should be consulted regarding your specific situation.

Library of Congress Cataloging-in-Publication Data:

Farr, Mary I.
  The heart of health : embracing life with your mind and spirit /
Mary I. Farr.
     p.   cm.
   ISBN 0-471-34803-1 (pbk. : alk. paper)
   1. Health—Philosophy. 2. Health—Religious aspects.
 3. Spiritual life. 4. Mind and body. 5. Healing—Religious
 aspects. I. Title.
 RA776.5.F36   2000
 610'.1—dc21   99-33637

Printed in the United States of America

10 9 8 7 6 5 4 3 2 1

For Andra and Christian

Contents

Acknowledgments

The stories you are about to read reveal the kind of truths discovered in the lives of real people. Though I have adjusted names and details to protect an individual's privacy, each chapter reflects a measure of wisdom that originates with ordinary people living their lives with extraordinary spirit. I wish to express my gratitude to each of these individuals, especially the families, children, and gifted health care providers I have come to know in my work as a hospital chaplain at Children's Hospitals and Clinics in St. Paul, Minnesota. Accompanying them through joyful and immeasurably difficult life events has been both a privilege and a blessing.

The Heart of Health

Listening Means Everything When It Comes to Health

※⸙

"No one listens," they tell me, and so I listen . . . and I tell them what they have just told me, and I sit in silence, listening to them, letting them grieve. "Julian, you are wise," they say. "You have been gifted with understanding." And all I did was listen, for I believe full surely that God's spirit is in us all.

—Julian of Norwich,
Thirteenth-century English mystic

LISTENING LIES at the very heart of medicine. It also lies at the heart of justice, love, and peace. Our need to listen is surpassed only by our need to connect with one another and walk together on the holy ground of our human experience. *The Heart of Health* is a book about listening and connecting. It is a book with a message for anyone who has ever experienced illness or loss, practiced medicine, or educated a health care professional.

With an eye to defining health, the following stories invite readers to take seriously the meaning of wholeness in their lives and in the lives of those they care for. Meaning, after all, is as valuable as knowledge in understanding health. Though the pursuit of scientific knowledge continues to supply today's medical practitioners with extraordinary tools for diagnosing and curing, it is meaning that changes one's experience of life and health. While Western biomedicine pursues more technology and treatment, fatigue, numbness, and overwork impair health professionals at an alarming rate. Doctors struggle to advocate for their patients in ten-minute increments. Families feeling isolated and alone search the Internet for more compassionate treatment alternatives. On a bad day, health care reveals precious little evidence of health or care.

In fact, years of working with children, families, and other caregivers have shown me that health involves much more than repaired body systems, and that healing happens at the level of soul. And when people ask me, "Where is God in today's newspaper reports of violence and apathy?" or "What is God's role in sickness and death?" my answer can only be that the God I know is right here, in the faces and hands of those we encounter every day. The faith I embrace does not consist of a belief that we will be rescued from disease or death. It consists of a belief that we are loved, and that no amount of suffering or illness can diminish our value and purpose in this world. The life of each of us is incredibly important. We share that message every time we choose to show up, listen, and speak the truth. Each of us has a story to tell as well as a need to listen—especially when it comes to being well. This is true whether we are at the giving or receiving end of care.

Sixteen-year-old Kevin, who comes to terms with an aggressive brain tumor; your neighbor forced to retire early with a debilitating back injury—both know that treating and curing are often impossible and always inadequate. As friends and companions on the journey, we must also walk with one another when cure eludes us. Developing this inner sensitivity gives birth to the beginning of our own spiritual lives. It also redefines our roles as ones of service to others, service we offer by creating a space in which another can heal. By making room in our hearts to receive another's story, we learn more about his or her health and we learn to listen to our own inner voice. By restoring our sense of service to humanity, we begin to draw from a place of abundance and hope and to share that energy with those who hunger for it. I have discovered that by insisting on the need for both hearing another and embracing the idea of service, we can breathe life back into the alarmingly brittle soul of today's health care culture.

Meanwhile, those of us seeking to live a life of wholeness must also look to our spiritual selves as having a role in defining health. Our spiritual lives, after all, arise from our human lives. For example, the way we live, care for our physical bodies, and interpret the mystery that surrounds us informs our health. So, too, do the ways we celebrate our joys and find support in our pain, conflicts, and losses; the way we nurture and shepherd our children; and the way we respond to and protect the earth and her resources. Spiritual issues such as these deeply affect our sense of well-being. Our capacity for healing directly reflects our capacity for drawing from our inner life of spirit. Our neglect of that inner life places us in greater danger of ill health.

History tells us that humankind once understood health as a state of wholeness extending far beyond fixing and curing disease. Many ancient traditions offer a rich history of healing rooted not just in the natural sciences but in the essence of our humanity—in our senses. Holistic traditions such as these recognized both the curative power of nutrition and the healing capacity of the rituals and aromas of "breaking bread" together. Health as viewed from this broader perspective also affirmed the healing value of spirituality and prayer . . . of relationships . . . of community and the support of others . . . of love . . . of healing touch . . . of reconciliation and letting go . . . and of saying good-bye. Somehow, in the course of only a few decades, however, we seem to have forgotten these essential elements of healing. Somehow, we seem to have forgotten even the true meaning of health.

Simultaneously, a growing interest in alternative medicine has begun to reveal another aspect of health and health care today—the changing role of physicians. Once shamans and healers immersed in the daily lives of their communities, doctors have evolved into clinical practitioners hamstrung by a new vocabulary of clinical standards, quality control, and customer service. We have veered away from the idea of physician as healing companion; medicine is now understood as a vast development of the natural sciences and as the application of physics, chemistry, and mathematics to the study of life processes. Doctors trained and encouraged to adopt an engineer's approach to health have found themselves tackling illness as if it were mechanical trouble and turning medical therapy into little more than technical manipulation. Clearly this brave new physician role has helped in the correct diagnosis and treatment of countless medical conditions. Yet just as clearly, this role, having left behind so much, has found many doctors wondering why they chose to practice medicine, and many patients wondering how to find healing.

This is a book about doctors and patients coming of age. It's about families and caregivers and exploring the wider boundaries of healing—about a deeper understanding of human health. Perhaps health care's pendulum must reach its highest technological point before beginning a life-giving swing toward fruitful integration with other aspects of the human person and other healing traditions. *The Heart of Health* contends that society and health care, trapped in their high-tech prison—with its Internet and e-mail avoidance of personal contact and relationships—have lost sight of the healing essences that make us human.

We've learned a lot that should help us rethink the way we look at health. We know, for instance, that health is not merely the absence of disease, and that purely scientific medicine is simply not sufficient for our needs or the needs of the people we care for. We know, too, that people want scientific medicine yet long for other dimensions of healing. Both doctors and patients have expressed to me their yearning for answers that offer comfort, relief, restoration, and healing beyond cure. I've listened to both doctors and patients express the same longing to have meaningful relationships with one another. *The Heart of Health* not only assumes that this integration is possible but also offers timely and practical information that will help healers and their patients understand the sum of conventional and ancient understandings of health. Through a blend of patient, family, and physician stories, the book helps define health in its fullest measure.

Readers gain a picture of health shaped by qualities such as the strength of a human spirit, the therapeutic value of community, and the healing essence of compassion. Chapters consist of personal vignettes, parables, and even recipes that suggest simple ways by which we all might preserve and protect our health and the health of our families and loved ones . . . even when cure is no longer the goal. Essential questions begin to emerge from these chapters about how we live and work, how we cope with the many health-denying elements of contemporary culture, and what doctors and patients can realistically expect from one another.

The Heart of Health means to inspire and educate. It explores the role of spirituality in medicine from the perspectives of both patients and physicians, while it raises the issue of caring as a "vocation" that fosters health in oneself and others. Readers can expect to learn about spiritual, physical, and emotional components of health and illness. Discussion questions and personal inventories highlight self-care, while clarifying the difference between cure and healing and demonstrating that each of us can bring healing gifts to a different health condition.

Ultimately, this is a book about hope. I urge that we adopt a new stance of life in health care, a stance that invites attentive listening, remembering, and acting with justice. For even in the face of illness and death, life emerges. Even when we can see no reason for optimism, we can find reason for hope.

CHAPTER 1

Health Means Different Things to Different People

⊰⊱

Salus: (Latin) salvation or health
Salud: a toast, "to your health"

SEVERAL YEARS AGO, those of us who work with patients and families in the hospital where I am employed received a surprising assignment from our organization's leadership. We were asked to create an advertisement that told people about our work and how it affected the health of patients and their families. A successful ad had to clearly explain our services to a complete stranger in the time it took to ride the hospital elevator from the first floor to the fourth. What began as an entertaining, if not impossible, game among colleagues resulted in our deeper understanding of ourselves. It also taught us a good deal about the role of pastoral counseling, or soul care, in healing.

It seemed no small paradox that, though we chaplains worked in a thoroughly modern health care facility, we offered no conventional health care tools—no clear-cut methods of diagnosing illness, no lifesaving technology, surgery, or scientific research, no prescriptions, no cures. We generated no revenue, nor did we provide any clinical model for measuring the quality

7

or cost-effectiveness of our work. By today's measures and efficiency standards, we held an indefensible position in a health care
institution. Stranger still, we often earned high family-satisfaction
marks in situations where a child suffered a serious health crisis
or even died. I might add, however, that we chaplains also view
health through a very different lens from that used by many
health care professionals and even patients. Instead of curing
ailments, we offer safe space in which others can consider the
possibility of being well or whole. This book highlights many of
the truths we see through that lens.

The care of the soul, or the act of shepherding the inner life
of people, reveals profound information about the meaning of
health. Through the years, I've learned that caring for the soul
of someone who wrestles with the consequences of illness dis-
closes important stories that can be helpful for patients and
their caregivers alike. Soul care touches subjects such as hopelessness and loss, while science, for its part, continues to produce indisputable evidence about body systems and restoring
health. It seems to me that matters of the human mind and
spirit contribute equally to the idea of health and to health
itself.

For example, an elderly man living in his own home might
tell me that mobility, independence, and family connections
mean everything to him—they come to mind first when he
thinks about good health. That same man would probably view
confinement, loneliness, and isolation as aspects of ill health.
Health observed from a spiritual perspective encompasses all
of these, plus the quality of our celebrations and the measure
of our gratitude. It also encompasses the way we process grief,
and our experience of intimacy with others. Good health, it
seems, is often accompanied by a willingness to receive life in its
entirety as fundamentally acceptable. It's about finding peace of
mind in an imperfect, ambiguous world. While health viewed in
this manner does not promise a life without suffering, those

who enjoy good health tend to embrace an expectation of future good—a fundamental posture of gratitude and reconciliation.

Health and wholeness, then, point to the idea that we are human, with human limitations. Though science and biomedicine continue to advance the preservation and repair of biological health, many more personal aspects of our lives predict our capacity for wholeness; these are the things for which our hearts and bodies most yearn.

CHAPTER 2

Science Tells Us Many Things but Not the Meaning of Health

❧✦❧

Dramatic advances in the prevention and treatment of life-threatening illnesses have dazzled us during the past century. Science continues to produce medical triumphs in diagnosis, surgery, and drug therapy. Organ repair and replacement, restoration of hearing and sight, cures of many types of cancer and long-term arrest of others—these only begin the list of modern medicine's achievements. Something is missing, however. Conspicuously absent in this medical success story is a basic understanding of the meaning of health. Proof of this emerged the first time I asked a group of medical residents in our hospital to tell me about health and illness. Nobody had much to say, nor had they spent much time in medical school covering this topic.

Treatments and cures abound, yet the residents acknowledged that many of their patients in clinic did not respond to drug therapy, surgery, or other treatments. Other patients—especially those who had left other cultures to come to the United States—often reached out for medical help when they really suffered from sorrow and self-limiting disorders well

within the range of their body's own healing powers. Simultaneously, many of the residents reported their own struggles with
losses, exhaustion, and a prevailing sense of the bleakness of
life. It seemed that countless anxiety-producing issues associated with their training contributed to their quiet despair, to
their need to be heard, perhaps to their dis-ease. All of these
conditions have to do with health, yet none responds well to
today's model of health care.

Western medicine, with its strictly scientific approach, has
considered health only in anatomical or physiological terms,
as a matter of human parts subdivided down to the smallest
observable detail. For all that can be observed, however, many
qualities of health are less observable. For all that science has
achieved, it has neglected the whole picture of human health, a
picture far greater than the sum of its parts.

This model of treating disease and defining health offers little to parents wrestling with the losses surrounding their child's
brain tumor. Nor does it hold much consolation for the
anguished teenager with anorexia nervosa, or for the burned-
out medical resident who doubts everything from her professional judgment to her life choices. Finally, this model of care
does not have time to recognize that although people want and
need scientific medicine, they hunger for other dimensions of
healing. I believe they are searching for a new (or perhaps
ancient) understanding of "shalom."

In the Judeo-Christian tradition, the word for peace is shalom. We experience shalom as an act of God's graciousness in
our lives. Such peace is more than simply an absence of conflict;
"shalom" really means wholeness. It plays a vital role in building and protecting the well-being of all our communities including our families, our neighborhoods, and our workplaces.

To greet someone with "shalom" is to ask, "How is it with
you? Do you have work? Does your family have enough food?
Do you have adequate shelter?" It implies that the one who asks

the question accepts some level of responsibility for the other person's well-being. We offer this gift of shalom to one another in many ordinary ways—by listening and affirming and by our acts of goodwill.

Shalom points to the idea of being well. Similarly, the terms "cure" and "healing" reflect two distinct avenues to the same end: becoming well. Used in this context, "cure" refers primarily to specific acts of scientific intervention. These interventions could consist of surgery, the taking of prescription drugs, and the application of technology.

"Healing," on the other hand, points to a set of possibilities that everyone, especially health care professionals, can bring to a seemingly incurable situation. While a healing approach may not always change a medical outcome or control social and environmental problems, it can positively affect our own and others' health. A healing approach encompasses assets that all of us—physicians, nurses, family, friends, and colleagues—already possess. When we choose to offer these assets to others, we foster their feelings of safety, wholeness, and hope. Sharing these assets also tends to create in us a sense of belonging and of being connected to one another.

If cure cannot be separated from healing, neither can healing be disconnected from shalom. Each of us contributes immeasurably to this totality called health by promoting the following aspects of peace and healing: hospitality; presence; listening; compassion; advocacy; acceptance; hope; and gratitude.

CHAPTER 3

Scientific Medicine Has Many Answers . . . Not All

~⊛⊛~

A DOCTOR AND A PATIENT bring quite different tools to the project of building health. The doctor comes with prescriptions, surgery, and a host of medical manipulations that cure. The patient brings the potential for healing.

Today's growing interest in the human soul arises because science and medicine have simply not given us all the answers to good health. In fact, when serious illness strikes, I've watched it set off a chain of events that touch every aspect of a person's life. Sickness and human suffering are a shattering occurrence that can cause everything from broken relationships to bankruptcy. I once had a woman tell me she had decided to buy an expensive dress to wear to her child's funeral because her family was already so financially devastated that the added cost would hardly cause a ripple. For someone who is ill, or for a parent of a dying child, it is vital to seek good care as well as to make sense of the illness. Just as important is the search for meaning and hope in life and in saying good-bye to life.

Patients and loved ones often express concern about the condition of health care today. Why do they pursue questionable therapies or put their hopes in undocumented research instead of visiting with their own doctors to discuss their options? The answer: Their sense of brokenness amounts to much more than damaged body parts. Wholeness does not just happen through compartmentalizing the human body, as in conventional medicine, but through attending to a person's comfort and peace as well. For instance, to ask a woman with diabetes about her symptoms is an important question for her doctor. But it is equally important to ask that same person what it means to live with diabetes.

Patients and doctors both worry about today's increased emphasis on productivity, efficiency, and cost containment in health care. They complain of feeling like numbers in a corporate health care world. Yet, numbers and measures aside, at the heart of every illness lies a human need for connection and intimacy. This may not sound like efficient business or objective science, but it says volumes about health.

Add to patients' fears of anonymity the fact that modern medicine has become overly concerned with correct diagnosis and with defining health solely in physiological terms. Hospitals, meanwhile, have evolved into places of business whose primary purpose is to generate income by curing diseases in the shortest possible time. Both these factors drive people to search more deeply, stretching their boundaries—and sometimes losing their good judgment—as they seek healing.

Finally, many people today are discovering pieces of a long historical relationship between medicine and religion, a relationship that begs to be renewed. Indeed, it is the two together, not in isolation, that furnish the foundation for good health.

HOSPITALITY *The act of offering hospitality to another is an act of graciousness; to be hospitable is to be receptive, helpful, generous, benevolent, courteous, and neighborly in response to others. Hospitality begins in the human heart and consists of simple acts of courtesy that provide comfort and consolation. A hospitable heart is a heart that can make room for another's story.*

CHAPTER 4

First, We Must Make a Commitment to Care

⟡

A PHYSIOLOGIST whose research focused on the human heart once offered me a provocative piece of information. "When you place cells from two separate hearts into a single incubating medium, they begin to communicate with one another," he said. It seems that certain proteins in heart-cell membranes enable the cells to communicate with one another. Unlike other body cells, those that make up the human heart can transfer electrical energy from cell to cell. Once placed in a petri dish, the faster-beating cells tell the slower-beating cells to speed up until, eventually, the two kinds beat in unison. As one. Compelling evidence that, at the very center of our being, we humans are quite literally connected.

Ancient and primitive societies have always had effective healers who understood this phenomenon at a spiritual, rather than scientific, level. For millennia, science played an unimportant role in medical care. Most ancient societies based nearly all of their medical procedures on religious belief, cultural values, and crude empiricism. Ancient Egypt furnishes the earliest recorded history of a highly developed practice of medicine, in which physician-priests ensured that medicine remained closely associated with religion. Priests and laypeople believed that disease and death were by-products of evil influences working through visible or invisible agents of destruction. The cures that overthrew these agents found their power in magic, spells, and prayers.

The Babylonians and Assyrians introduced astrology into medicine; Greek civilization rooted medicine more firmly in a process of observation. Greece also produced dualisms—spirit over body, mind over matter—that have had a lasting influence on medicine.

With Hippocrates, who was born around 460 B.C., came the flowering of Greek medicine. Hippocrates and his contemporaries offered natural rather than supernatural explanations of illness and based these explanations on observation.

Christianity emphasized the healing miracles of Jesus Christ; healing of the body was one with healing of the mind and spirit. The church turned away from the ancients' focus on the powers of nature, and looked toward God as the source of nature itself.

Around the sixteenth century, the pace of medical science accelerated, and that acceleration has continued ever since. From the seventeenth century onward, the destinies of medicine entered into an inseparable association with those of the natural sciences.

By the end of the nineteenth century, Cartesian and Newtonian models of the universe and its underlying reality were firmly in place. Newton's physics and mathematics led him to describe the universe as a great cosmic machine. Humans could understand this machine by breaking it down and analyzing its parts.

Most of the dramatic advances of medicine in the last century have also resulted from the breakdown and analysis of component parts, through the tremendous development of natural sciences and the application of physics, chemistry, and mathematics to the study of life processes. Only in the last century has it become usual to think of authentic medical practice as limited to surgery and drugs.

As a by-product of the strictly scientific approach to medicine that evolved in the nineteenth century, the sphere of the responsible healer became more confined to the definition and treatment of ill health of the human body. Our concept of matter over mind continues to influence all of us, from nursery school onward. We learn to become objective and detached when solving problems. We learn to observe, analyze, and record data. Given this history, it's not surprising that we have difficulty entering into a subjective personal or spiritual experience and then accepting that experience as valid.

Within this model of thought, the spiritual and cultural elements of human illness became suspect. They cannot so easily be touched or observed, nor can we measure their impact. When human problems land outside secure scientific footing, they seem not to exist, or at least seem to lack a certain degree of authenticity. In this climate, patients can unintentionally become diagnostic problems and death a medical failure that somehow escaped a logical solution. And people who suffer with problems such as apathy or chronic anxiety quickly learn they need to get hold of themselves and get over it.

Taken to the extreme, this approach defines health as only the absence of disease, and illness as a technical malfunction requiring mechanical adjustment or a quick prescription fix. Medicine, even alternative medicine, still tends to direct its attention toward curing the body rather than toward healing the person.

All this places the heart-tissue I described earlier in an ironic light. The science that continues to produce advances in medicine; the science that finds its success through breaking down and analyzing parts; the science that thrives on objective observation and tangible evidence is the same science that now shows us a powerfully religious notion: our actual connection to one another.

This irony came to mind when a nurse manager in the pediatric hospital where I work appeared at my office door asking if she could talk. "I have no idea what's happened to my staff," she announced, "but I do know we have to do something about it . . . now."

The woman proceeded to tick off a catalog of disturbing attitudes and behaviors exhibited by her employees: Anxiety. Anger. Depression. Rigidity. Self-righteousness. Intolerance. Absenteeism. Their individual demands and grievances had grown to the point of choking out their esprit de corps. Indifferent nurses demonstrated only marginal levels of courtesy and good spirit, shuffled through their daily tasks, and departed for home as quickly as possible.

This raised particular concern. Generally, those who choose to work in health care, especially children's health care, choose it with a sense of altruism. Hospital departments and nursing units usually become very close, even functioning as extended families.

True, our hospital's recent merger with another pediatric facility had probably given rise to some of the sourness. With change as a new paradigm in the health care world, we all felt added pressure to perform better with less. Most in leadership positions anticipated tension and tried to prepare themselves and their staffs for the roiling waters of consolidation. Lost jobs, new jobs, blended work cultures—the hospital was destined to be a difficult place for a while.

The manager and I concluded that we would gather some information from others in the hospital and then reconvene to compare notes and make a plan. I didn't have to look far. Others spontaneously came to my office to express their concern. They arrived from the hospital emergency department and the pediatric intensive care unit. A vice president called. A psychologist and several physicians asked to meet. Entire nursing units requested that our chaplains take part in their retreats and department meetings, trying to get at the source of their angst. Their stories resembled the nurse manager's. It seemed that we faced a problem larger than department integration or patient care redesign. We were suffering from a health crisis of a different nature, one that often occurs when people feel they have lost control of their lives and nobody cares.

The diagnosis that began to take shape was of spiritual malaise sparked by a prickly business transition. Throughout the hospital, staff reported feelings of disharmony and grief at losing old relationships and routines. Many complained of feeling unappreciated and nameless.

While a children's hospital might seem like a specialized institution with specialized employee needs, I'm convinced that those with whom I interact daily represent much more than a health care institution. They speak for a world of others who get up each day feeling half-sick at having to face their workplace. Their anxiety resembles that of countless others. Their need for friendship, kinship, and meaningful work is shared by all of us. Their desire to feel grounded and valued reflects everyone's hope for the same. And these needs and desires all shape our state of health or lack of it.

So, what's missing? How can we feel complete and well? What have we lost in our communities? What's become of our businesses and institutions, which once felt like communities and now leave us feeling like exiles? And how do we begin to quench this human thirst to be part of a worthwhile plan and a larger whole?

We began to raise these questions among other managers and hospital administrators. A few resisted, suggesting that what people really needed to do was stop whining and get on with things. "We live in a new world," they insisted, "and people had better get used to it."

Some months later, armed with more complete information and some encouragement from all the staff, our hospital administration retained a group of consultants who spent the next two years helping us examine ourselves as a community of caregivers. What began with a small group of concerned employees grew into a comprehensive study of our work environment. During that time, we learned a great deal about health that had little to do with medicine. I'm certain that this important adventure will serve us all well in the future.

Themes took shape. While some dealt with job function and process, others spoke of spiritual concerns. For example, fear of losing jobs and of facing an unknown future ran high. Frustrations led to a sense of powerlessness. Feelings of being lost in a large, corporate environment led people to believe they had no influence over organizational decisions. Many employees described symptoms of grief. Interestingly, most of the emotions we identified among the people we interviewed mirrored those of the patients and families who came to our hospital.

The larger picture continues to unfold. Long-term solutions could eventually include everything from architectural alterations that encourage more personal contact to cultural awareness education, festive occasions, and more money for professional development. Many of our chaplain staff consciously apply spiritual principles that we know foster healing. Everyone we encounter in our hospital—every nurse, doctor, administrator, cook, and housekeeper—finds us advocating the same principles we have advocated with patients and families for years:

Make a space for others.
Invite them to tell their story.
Listen.
Help them identify ways, however small, to put order to
    or gain control over their lives.
Simplify our work.
Encourage one another.
Affirm colleagues as well as patients.
Permit grief.

So, after all the meetings have ended and the consultants have returned to their offices, after all the quality assurance measures and benchmarks have been replaced by new ones, our mission as health care providers and colleagues comes down to just one thing—we simply cannot fail when we choose to care for one another.

We belong to families of countless stars . . .

CHAPTER 5

Belonging Fosters Well-Being

❧❦

Belong: to have a proper or suitable place; to be part of, related to, or connected to; to be a member of.

Everyone wants to belong. Everyone *needs* to belong.

We belong to families of countless shapes and sizes. We belong to churches, support groups, work groups, book clubs, and professional organizations. Most certainly we all know what it feels like to belong. Or do we?

Sixteen years have passed since I formally took up a vocation of listening to people talk about their lives—their dreams, their losses, their unmet needs. For a hospital chaplain and teacher, attending to the human story means everything. The stories I hear every day speak of sickness and health. They describe success and failure, recovery and death. They touch every possibility, and a few impossibilities, that folks carry with them when they arrive at our hospital door. They embrace virtually every social, economic, and cultural experience one can imagine. Yet, while these stories differ widely in their circumstances, often they share a theme: the problem of belonging—or, perhaps more accurately, of not belonging.

Hospitals, in my experience, have always felt like small worlds of their own populated by close-knit health care workers whose lives merge with the lives of patients of every description. Maybe this is because hospitals contain the full measure of life's drama under one roof, from birth to death, sickness to health, and all manner of socioeconomic dilemmas. What I do know is that day in and day out, the entire range of human behavior flows through the hallways and nursing units, enacted by everyone from housekeepers to surgeons. I'm convinced that hospitals reflect quite accurately the mood of our larger society; if so, then Americans everywhere suffer from an eroded sense of belonging. And belonging, I've learned, is a primary aspect of good health.

I see several societal shifts contributing to this decreased feeling of belonging. A culture of shifting landscapes and diminishing guideposts has translated to a climate of chronic insecurity. We feel ambivalent about our work. We try to adjust to our persistent anxiousness. We find ourselves looking deeply into our own stories for signs and direction. Where are we? Do we even have the capacity to feel "a part of"? Do we possess the resources to connect deeply with one another, or must we go looking for them?

The answer, I believe, is yes, we do have the resources. No, we do not have to look beyond ourselves for them. However, to tap the wellspring of intimacy we require commitment, nurture, and maybe even a change of heart. There are simply no quick fixes and no easy answers to fill this need of belonging. Ultimately there is no path but the path made by our own walking. Part of the way to belonging lies in our capacity to rediscover our humanity and our inherent human skill to be our brother's keeper. Through this, we learn about our extraordinary ability to create a sense of place for ourselves. We begin to see everyday experiences and relationships in new ways, as rich sources of vitality and sustenance.

Belonging takes work. It sometimes means refashioning our communities on the job and at home, or at least rediscovering the value of wasting time wisely with those we care about. It means including those who are alone. To belong is to move in the direction of the larger whole, not simply toward our own goals and objectives. Belonging invites well-being or, to put it another way, being well.

CHAPTER 6

Not Belonging Invites
Isolation and Loneliness

❦

*Persons who are socially isolated often visit physicians
because they do not feel cared for, valued or esteemed.
They seek advice, interpersonal stimulation and the sense
of belonging and sustenance that a social support system
provides.*

—Arthur Barsky

YEARS AGO my brother convinced my parents to celebrate
Christmas on Christmas Eve. (In previous years, we'd opened
gifts and enjoyed our festive meal on Christmas Day.) If I'm not
mistaken, my mother also tampered with the menu that year,
substituting jellied cranberry sauce for the whole berries. In
fact, she might have placed the tree in a different location to free
the living room so that we could use the fireplace.

For the next decade, every member of our family talked
about the year my mother ruined Christmas. A woman who had
never intentionally done an unkind thing had dared to change a
few old traditions, not even particularly good ones. Nobody was
about to let her forget her indiscretion.

Change, especially changing the way we've always done
things, troubles most of us. Change can be as simple as adjusting

to daylight saving time or as complex as gaining a new perspective on racial or political matters. In any case, change threatens to destroy the shield that protects our security. It sends up red flags of discomfort and leaves us feeling faintly unsettled or, in some cases, paralyzed. But change can often point us toward a new doorway to wholeness. Our ability or lack of ability to alter attitudes and routines determines the quality of everything from our careers to our personal relationships, from our problem-solving skills to our spiritual growth.

I'm convinced that few of us actually *choose* to change much. Instead, we tend to move, somewhat grudgingly, with the flow, making necessary adjustments along the way. Rarely do we resist like the woman I know who simply said no, and then retreated to an empty house on a remote hilltop. At ninety-four, she still has no intention of changing anything, including her cloistered lifestyle. Living with other people would require more adjustments than she is willing to make. Instead, she has chosen a life of isolation.

Florence Sedgwick lives in the hills of western Wisconsin. Over the decades, she withdrew from her small farming community. Only an occasional bit of gossip reminds local residents that she ever lived there. Jason Bauer in the Mondovi Co-op Equity claimed she buried a fortune under her hay shed. A butcher in Bob's IGA insisted that she was once committed to a mental institution. A World War I veteran in the local nursing home said she set fire to a bunkhouse up the valley on the Werlein farm, a fire that killed her supposedly philandering husband. Nevertheless, after years of speculation, nobody really knew much about Florence, or Flossie, as she chose to be called. All this struck me as curious, because the ramshackle, unpainted fortress where she lived was only a few miles west of town.

No photos or records of her existed in the local library. No letters or church archives held a reliable history of her. The unkempt footpath leading to her front door testified that nobody came to call. She lived a solitary existence, a hermit who aroused only a modest ripple of curiosity. A few enterprising journalists once tried to interview her for a feature in the local newspaper, but they found themselves looking down the business end of a twelve-gauge shotgun. To the best of everyone's knowledge, they never went back.

Concerning the mysterious space of her hermitage, the bizarre tales proliferated. Hence, I seriously questioned my judgment on that June morning when I rode my horse up the lane to her house. The early sun slanted through an old apple orchard, the trees like broken sentries guarding the entrance to her property. A first cutting of hay lay in damp windrows beneath the ground fog. Cows and their calves traversed the hillside to rejoin one another after a night spent scattered throughout the pasture. We passed an abandoned cottage where O'Malley's hired man, Mel Jacobson, used to live. The cats had taken charge ever since Mel had a stroke and moved to the Valley Nursing Home in Durand. A litter of kittens tumbled off the front stoop into a neglected bed of daylilies.

I might not have seen her if she hadn't frightened my horse, causing him to vault up an embankment. By anybody's standards, she was an awesome sight, a wizened gnome stooped in the tall grass. She clutched the handle of a double-bladed ax. Her expression hovered between anger and interest. She crouched, poised for combat. Oddly, she wore a dress. Odder still, the dress was secured with large safety pins to several layers of long underwear. Her leathery skin hung about her neck and over her muscular arms. She had immense hands that looked as if they belonged to a man. A pink plastic barrette held her hair off her forehead, and a plain wedding band and wire-rimmed spectacles offered the only clues that she had ever known human contact.

My horse was by now hopelessly unmanageable; I had to dismount or be thrown. Choosing the first option, I slipped out of the saddle and stood about a dozen feet from the old woman. She gripped her ax but didn't make any threatening moves, nor did she run away. A long moment passed before it occurred to me to offer my hand in a greeting. Surprisingly, she stepped forward, shook my extended hand, and began to talk about my horse's behavior.

"I'm not surprised he's afeared of me," she announced simply. "Dogs is, too. It's because I'm too old. I've lived too long. But my cat Jefferson back home . . . well, now, that's a different story. He loves me. Never leaves home for longer than a day. He stays to home the way he should."

I soon learned that Flossie was born on a small farm in the nearby township of Dover. "Three generations of us have growed up right in this here area," she explained. "My mother was born in a log cabin on the hill behind my place. This is home for me. I'd rather take a pounding than go to town. As far as I'm concerned, I'll be here on my forty three hundred and sixty-five days a year till the day I die."

Eccentric or not, Flossie had something in common with any of us who ever wanted to run away from the pain and responsibility of living with others. The primary difference in Flossie was that she never mastered the art of adapting to change. The losses and setbacks that most people experience in a lifetime drove her in a different direction. Through the years, she slowly withdrew, finally choosing to make her journey alone rather than risk any more losses or adjustments.

Flossie and her husband, "the Old Gent," began farming their plot in 1920. "We worked with the neighbors back then," she said, "especially when we were threshing or shredding. I had my own beautiful team, Florie Bay and Ted. Them and me hauled grain shocks out of the field all day long. After the bundles dried, I'd run the steam thresher to separate the grain from the straw. I've never driven a car, but I can drive any horse or steam engine you could find me."

Flossie chose her own road and then walked it . . . alone. As she groped through her memories of cooking and harvesting, I could see how each bit of past misfortune had nudged her further from the company of others. During our subsequent visits, she stitched for me a patchwork account of her history: the Depression; crop losses and the Old Gent's death; her children leaving home; automated methods of farming; a legal battle to keep her beloved forty. Faced with seemingly endless difficult decisions, she focused on the only thing she felt she had left— her homestead. "I made up my mind long ago I would rally here or perish," she said. "It's quiet here and it's mine."

There she remained, spending most of her hours collecting fruits and nuts, chopping brush and splitting firewood for her Heaterolla stove. Every summer a local mill delivers ten loads of wood. By fall, she has cut and neatly stacked each piece behind her back porch. Now and then, someone drops off food and other staples at her mailbox. She loads the supplies into a wheelbarrow and pushes it up the half-mile hill. Jars of canned meats and fruits fill her pantry shelf, and large bowls of hand-pumped water line the countertop. Rags curtain the open windows, and braided rugs are scattered on the unfinished wood floor. In a wooden crate next to the pump house sleeps her companion, Jefferson.

Flossie's story was both troubling and seductive. I saw something deliciously alluring about the idea of vanishing, of casting off the complicated relationships and demanding commitments that sap me of energy. Nevertheless, Flossie also bore the unmistakable signs of estrangement and sadness that accompany a choice to retreat. Though she spoke with enthusiasm about her life on the forty, I sensed a hollowness in her spirit and a longing for human contact that had nothing to do with age.

Most of the locals were satisfied to call Flossie crazy, but her desire to escape is far from unique. Scores of people race through life, paying it little more than a courtesy call; they're visitors and sightseers instead of pilgrims. Consider how many friends who are injured by divorce never choose intimacy again. Think of those who remain stuck in insufferable jobs and abusive relationships. The fact is, a large segment of the human race views success as something that comes only when we bolt down the hatches and secure all aspects of our lives into predictable patterns of sameness, efficiency, and stability.

Success as I've grown to understand it cannot be measured by what one is or does, but only by distance traveled. We are forever moving from one experience to another, one challenge to another, one relationship, one loss or achievement to another. We are unfinished business, shaped and reshaped by our continuing experience. It is this fluid and changing quality of life that invites us to become resilient rather than resistant, to belong rather than to retreat. Openness and a receptive heart clear the way for more adventure. To be open means to make ourselves available to life. Openness allows us to drop our past rebuffs and rejections, our victories and our failures. It helps us to see things afresh, as always newborn and stocked with possibilities. The challenge is to become so open to life that nothing can destroy us.

The ability to handle change and stay connected is a learned gift. It often demands many alterations in the original plan. These changes pull us out of our secure little niches and place us in unfamiliar territory. We instinctively want security, even if that security is an unpleasant repetition of past mistakes. The learning comes in letting go of some of the controls we tend to apply. The rewards come with discovering those things that we might have missed through our own refusal to consider a new way.

Nowhere are there any written guarantees that things will work out comfortably for us. Yet joy comes from our ability to transform and grow together with others in spite of discomfort and ambiguity. We gain nothing by pulling down the blinds or by giving way to cynicism and despair.

How sad it would be for us to go to the kitchen one morning and find there was no bread. How much more sad if we were to go to the kitchen and find that we weren't hungry.

CHAPTER 7

To Some, Health Is a Value Judgment

⤙✦⤚

A few years ago, I visited an old family friend, Ruth, who was enjoying her elder years on a lovely Wisconsin farm. Upon my arrival, she herded me outside for an agricultural and small-animal tour. We began with a brief hike to the edge of a small pond where I sat quietly and listened as she chatted with her granddaughter.

Three-year-old Christine squatted on top of an enormous rock pile, dabbling among her treasures of quartz and agate. Occasionally she tossed a small stone into the pond below, scattering a flock of Canada geese and their adolescent goslings. Four Bernese mountain dogs loped about the great mountain of stones, left over when the pond was dredged the previous spring. A chorus of joyful barks rained down upon the small child as she placidly sorted her treasure. The dogs—soaked, covered in sand—careened in and out of the water and around the older woman as she urged her granddaughter to come down and join her for a walk along the river. Ruth managed her home and her daily itinerary in a manner well suited to grandchildren and growing projects.

The driveway to her home revealed the first clues to Ruth's playful nature. A sign in front identified the small farm as the Shepherd's Patch, an allusion to her late husband, who was an

Episcopalian bishop. A flagpole served as the centerpiece of an indiscriminate array of toys, garden hoses, and unidentifiable items of clothing. The front porch, strewn with dog dishes, croquet mallets, and flats of petunias, provided a stage for children's productions. Clay pots filled with twigs and nuts lay among baking utensils and several hedge clippers. Two church pews, assorted cacti, and a wheelbarrow leaned against the garage. Hundreds of spotlessly cleaned dog bones mingled with decorative gravel, the only formal attempt at landscaping around the front porch. Spades, sprinkling cans, and pitchforks gave evidence of Ruth's interest in vegetable gardening and in her exquisite flock of Cotswold sheep.

The barn housed two Cotswold rams named Willie Billy and Billy Willie, more reminders of the dear departed "Very Reverend William." An old toolshed crammed with wire and stakes provided the backdrop for a dead pickup truck that listed gently over its front tires. A faded sign on the cow shed marked the property as a licensed game farm. Ruth hatched pheasant, fish, and waterfowl in cooperation with the Wisconsin Department of Natural Resources. It was her relationship with the DNR that prompted the pond-dredging project, which eventually produced hundreds of small trout and a swimming hole for the dogs.

Ruth's attire fluctuated throughout the day, from barn to garden to market apparel. That particular morning she wore a lemon-yellow T-shirt and blue knit pants. She also sported a baseball cap with an orange bird's-beak visor. Black patent-leather flats trimmed in multicolored buttons and floral print anklets completed her ensemble. She carried a grocery bag filled with asparagus that she and Christine had collected along the roadside. The combination of colors and sounds at the Shepherd's Patch reflected Ruth's unrestrained celebration of the simplest pleasures.

The word "celebration" usually implies music, dancing, and laughter—holidays and entertainments that help us temporarily forget the difficulties of life. We think of immersing ourselves in an atmosphere of pleasant unreality. But, from a more holistic perspective, celebration involves the acceptance of life and a constantly increasing awareness of its preciousness. Celebration happens only where fear and love, joy and sorrow, tears and smiles, young and old, can coexist with some measure of harmony. Life is precious, not only because it can be seen, touched, and tasted, but also because it will be gone one day.

Watching Ruth that morning, I saw a woman who had experienced her own losses and sorrows. Her husband had died a decade earlier. At age eighty-eight, she was entering her fifth year of trials and treatments for lymphoma. Lost bone density and the crippling effects of a deteriorated spine caused her significant pain. However, she continued choosing to live in the present and to go with whatever life handed her on that day. Christine and her other grandchildren invited her to be with them here and now. Their uninhibited expressions of affection and willingness to receive it pulled her directly into the moment and invited her to celebrate life where it could be found. Neither old age nor physical challenges would have caused her to say to her doctor that she was in "bad" health. Ruth had a strong community of family and friends and a genuine interest in others.

Today, five years later, Ruth continues to perk along. She still drives her car, much to her family's dismay—not because she can no longer rise to the challenges of driving, but because (according to them) she has driven outlandishly for some fifty years. Besides, her head barely reaches the top of the steering wheel. Once or twice a year she visits her older sister in California, tottering through airports alone and enjoying a little "change of venue." She is an avid reader and her nightstand sags under the weight of countless publications ranging from thrillers to the history of London. Each day finds her with a full schedule and an occasional nap—often in public or among friends who come to visit. Her spirit of discovery feeds her sense of whimsy and her confidence that "the fun is in the doing."

Knowing Ruth and many other elders who live with similar aspects of illness and old age, I began to consider health a matter of a value judgment—a judgment first made by a patient, but on which both physician and patient must ultimately agree. For example, an elderly woman might go to her physician's office with a daunting list of life-altering health conditions such as diabetes, glaucoma, and osteoarthritis. If that patient were Ruth, she probably would report to her physician that she was getting out and around, could do the things she enjoyed, and felt quite healthy.

Another woman of comparable age but with far fewer physiological problems might describe herself as quite ill and struggling with persistent pain and other life-restricting disabilities. The second patient, no doubt, would characterize herself as suffering from poor health. Both women would be telling the truth, though plainly they would see their health from quite different perspectives. In this case, their very real symptoms of good and ill health probably have less to do with organic problems than with their situation in life—their sense of connection with others, and their resilience. How they coped with life's accumulated losses might play a role in their perceptions of their own health. Family and social contacts also most likely would color both women's opinions about their own health. Each would make a value judgment about the quality of her health, a judgment modulated by many factors that reach deeper than conventional medicine.

Definitions of health abound, though most people would agree on certain basic elements. For example, good health includes an absence of significant disease and of excessive conflict, pain, or anxiety. Health also includes a sense of well-being, the ability to function effectively and in a reasonably good mood. A helpful definition of health also suggests a degree of self-discipline and balance, and it includes a capacity to love others and feel connected to them.

Illness, on the other hand, begins with the absence—partial or complete—of this valuable asset called health. The brokenness of illness involves threats to one's feelings of connection and meaning. Illness can interfere with a person's security, challenge her sense of control over her destiny, and produce feelings of alienation from her family, community, and God. Pain and loss of function disrupt one's ordinary means of making contact, thus intensifying detachment from everyday routines.

Like health, illness holds different meanings for different people. I've met patients and families who treated their illness as punishment or a sign of weakness or lack of faith. Others saw it as an enemy, to be fought with every weapon in the medical arsenal. For some, it became a strategy through which they manipulated others. And many saw illness as an irreparable loss or damage. In almost every case, the meaning of wellness or illness related directly to a person's perception of her or his life.

In addition to their physiological illness, many people have expressed to me their sense of the emptiness in our increasingly self-absorbed, secular culture. Violence, indifference, pollution, and other energy-depleting influences contribute to illness of a different nature. A need for all kinds of healing grows as more and more people lose their bearings. Many are searching for a new understanding of reality and a different structure of thought. It has become increasingly clear that the approach to health we've pursued for decades does not respond well to much of our ill health.

The past decade has found doctors and medical researchers paying more attention to the emotional and spiritual aspects of health. The roles of attitudes, emotions, and religious faith have become the subject of both research and practice at the most prestigious medical centers and schools, and the separation between secular and sacred, as well as that between the physical and the emotional, seems to be diminishing. Relaxation, mental imaging, and meditation are among the many techniques and therapies undergoing scientific testing to see if they change physical conditions. Researchers in the fields of psychoimmunology, psychology, neuroscience, and microbiology continue to confirm that the mind does influence the immune system.

Meanwhile, a growing body of evidence says we must broaden the base of medicine. Fundamental to both diagnosis and prognosis for a person complaining of ill health are many subtle, less tangible factors such as her or his emotional state and attitude toward the illness. Equally important is the therapeutic alliance between doctor and patient. These things are not new. Hippocrates long ago confirmed, "Some patients, though conscious that their condition is perilous, recover their health simply through their contentment with the goodness of the physician."[1]

In spite of the present movement toward a holistic approach to medicine, physicians feel pressured to control disease at all costs. The medical community in general, and hospitals in particular, tip the treatment scales in the direction of aggressive investigation, diagnosis, cure, and the prolongation of life at all costs. Patients continue to pressure doctors for a pain-free life and a quick fix. Even the incorporation of complementary or alternative therapies into today's medical treatment often assumes a cure-or-fix approach resembling the conventional medical approach that alternative practitioners hope to change.

In such a cure-oriented, death-defying environment, physicians and patients find it difficult to grasp the true essence of healing, which encompasses more than alleviating suffering (though it includes that). Healing and health are also about reconciliation. This reconciliation helps to engender wholeness. Genuine healing involves more than repairing or replacing damaged organs, more than eradicating disease. Genuine healing transcends physical repair and includes deep integration of body, mind, and spirit. This kind of healing suggests that patients do have self-corrective, innate, inward self-healing capacities.

Finally, to ask, "What does it mean to be healthy?" or "What does it mean to be healed?" is to ask a deeply religious question. Most seriously ill patients I have met eventually ask several predictable questions: "Why do I suffer?" "What does this illness mean?" "Why has God forsaken me?"

Women like Ruth have asked the same questions at some point along their course. Like others who find healing, she has discovered that the answers lie somewhere outside of science and technology . . . somewhere within themselves.

CHAPTER 8

Doctors Need to Remember Their Roles as Healers

❧❦

*Pythagoras said that the most divine art was that of heal-
ing. And if the healing art is most divine, it must occupy
itself with the soul as well as with the body; for no creature
can be sound as long as the higher part of it is sickly.*

—Apollonius of Tyana

ONCE I ASKED a group of pediatric residents to help me
understand the meaning of health. After a few halting attempts
at a definition, they retreated into silence. It became clear to all
of us that this topic had not made its way into their medical
school curriculums.

"Can you tell me why some patients with significant disease
say they are well, while others with no notable pathology say
they are sick?" I persisted.

A young woman then told us about her grandmother, a
feisty woman of ninety, who, to the amazement of everyone,
lived independently and in remarkably good health despite
having serious medical problems ranging from congestive heart

failure to macular degeneration. A discussion ensued, though only a few members of the group risked participating. We had stepped into what for most of them were uncharted waters.

But upon further consideration, the group agreed that health might be a subjective judgment that differed among individual patients and individual physicians. A healthy person typically enjoyed a high level of contentment and could function effectively in a reasonably good mood. The residents felt, too, that maintaining health required some kind of balance and self-responsibility. Further, most healthy adults they knew appeared to have a large capacity to love and forgive themselves and others. Finally, health seemed to thrive in the company of hope. With a little prodding, the fledgling physicians had opened the door to a larger view of health than they had thus far learned in medical school.

Illness, they then agreed, virtually always reached beyond the loss of health. Illness also presents patients and their families with a problem of meaning. Further, it often serves as a catalyst for many other disturbing events in their lives. A third-year neonatology fellow recalled how the parents of a very sick baby in our hospital's intensive care unit for newborns struggled to keep in touch with their friends. They finally set up a web site on their computer to tell others how their baby was progressing. He watched as they lost control of their lives and jobs while their infant languished in a tangle of monitors and IV lines. Their fears of being labeled "difficult" often kept these parents from complaining. At the same time, their own needs went unmet and their anxiety escalated. Disrupted routines and endless waiting placed terrible stress on their marriage.

The residents also observed that older children who came to the hospital experienced different kinds of losses related to their illnesses. Oncology patients undergoing chemotherapy faced painful loneliness. Separation from friends, an absence of social stimulation, and even the end of a sports career might follow a diagnosis of serious illness. Children often ask why they developed cancer. Did they do something wrong to cause their illness? How could they protect their parents from worrying about them? Social development, already a source of stress among young people, was made more painful by the prospect of returning to school with no hair.

Next, I asked the residents what they thought it meant to be a healer. Did they see the physician's role as that of a healer? If so, what would they need to be healers in today's health care environment?

"If my medical colleagues and I had been called healers, we wouldn't have known whether we were being praised or damned," says Larry Dossey, M.D., who writes about spirituality and medicine, and is former co-chair of the Panel on Mind/Body Interventions in the National Institutes of Health Office of Alternative Medicine.[1] Dossey observes that relatively little has changed since his medical education. "The concept of the healer remains virtually absent in medical training, and the term healing continues to be used in a narrow physiological sense," he explained.

According to Dossey, the medical profession's discomfort with healers and healing is an historical aberration. "For some 50,000 years, shamans and native healers of every variety have believed they possessed the powers to heal and were meant to be healers—convictions shared by their cultures."[2]

"Biomedicine" is the term applied to today's scientific medicine, which achieves medical advances by means of an increased understanding of the biological mechanisms of the body. The biomedical focus on a concept of matter over mind developed directly from the view of reality proposed by Descartes. By the middle of the twentieth century, the medical profession stood convinced that every something called a disease had something called a cure.

The biomedical approach has a firm base in the biological sciences. It has enormous technological resources at its command and a record of astonishing achievements in elucidating the mechanisms of disease and devising new techniques for treatment. While most health professionals recognize the tremendous value of a biomedical model of care, some advocate for expanding the model to recognize and attend to psychosocial factors in medical care.

For many health professionals, including the group of residents I spoke with, the concepts and practices at the heart of the only biomedical model remain firmly entrenched in their education. Few of the residents had had an opportunity to learn about the psychosocial issues in medicine. Medicine, for most of them, means concentrating on "real" diseases and avoiding the psychosocial underbrush. Practicing responsible medicine calls for disentangling the organic elements of disease from the social, emotional, and spiritual elements of human malfunctions. The implication persists that medicine wisely restricts itself to those elements of disease that can be explained in the language of physiology, biology, and ultimately biochemistry and physics, and that physicians are well advised to steer clear of problems that cannot be placed on the same securely scientific footing. Consequently, physicians still inclined to consider health and illness only in objective, scientific terms miss the opportunity to become healers.

One of the most difficult admissions for many physicians schooled in an era when the medical credo is to do and to cure is that of their own woundedness. In other words, to admit that they have no cure and to simply be with a patient armed only with their own stories and losses to the healing adventure seems like a medical failure. It has become more expedient to do something, sometimes anything. A clinician finds it extraordinarily difficult in today's clinical medicine to do what seems like nothing—for example, sitting quietly and attentively with a patient who has just received bad news. Doing nothing implies impotence and fallibility. The entire system teaches physicians that they do the curing, not that they serve as instruments through which curing comes as a gift. Such a system allows physicians to forget their own woundedness and potential sickness; it encourages arrogance.

The physician who struggles always to *do* has not yet learned that appropriate medical care is not something that someone does to another. It grows from the very essence of what a physician is. An authentic healer is willing to engage in a fearless personal evaluation of his or her inner state. Healers are not mechanics driving the patient's body to surgery or to the laboratory. Rather, they are persons who honor both the "human" and the "being" of the human being by becoming sensitive to the implicit order and rhythms of life.

When medical professionals act fully human, their actions produce fully appropriate decisions. However, in order to foster a fully human situation, a doctor must base her idea of patient care on a relationship of mutual respect and careful attentiveness. This relationship gains its substance from qualities such as mutuality, justice, balance, and compassion. The acceptance of individual freedom includes freedom for the physician to experience sorrow and kindheartedness, to take an inner stance of receptivity and offer an "I wish you well" attitude.

Medicine concerns itself with humankind. Science, for its part, sees only human parts. It is essentially analytical—that is to say, it divides and subdivides down to the tiniest detail. But for all it sees, it misses the whole picture, which is greater than the sum of its parts. A medical textbook produces descriptions of symptoms for every disease, but rarely will it include an appraisal of what disease is. It will describe every human organ and its function, but what is human it will not say. The things that pertain to wholeness exist beyond the eye of science. If one is to arrive at an understanding of the nature of human beings, of disease, of life, of healing, one must complement scientific knowledge, which is technical and analytical, with perspectives of a different, nonscientific order, the spiritual.

To advocate including the spiritual in healing is by no means to advocate a rejection of science. Yet the greatest scientists are the ones who understand that science has its limitations, too. "They know that two things go into the making of a doctor," said Swiss physician Paul Tournier, "great scientific competence and a great heart."[3]

Medical education within the present, restricted model cannot produce a great heart, nor can it even provide all the information a physician really needs. The ability to relate, to enter into contact with one's patients, to be open, to become a friend—this has nothing to do with science and must come from a different source. For today's young physicians to become healers, they must reintegrate those aspects of experience—body and mind, science and spirituality—that were divided so long ago. Only when the medical model includes the whole of a human being's experience can it guide clinicians toward their authentic role as healers, and help patients toward complete healing.

CHAPTER 9

The Doctor Who
Healed with Silence

❧❦

Simon, the son of Rabban Gamliel, said:
"I was brought up all my life among the Sages,
and I have found nothing as good for the body as silence,
and it is not study that is the essence—but the practice,
and whoever is profuse of words occasions sin."
—Pirke Avot 2:15, 16, *Sayings of Our Fathers*

Once, out of the blue, I received an invitation to write a speech for
a popular political figure. The address was to be given at an ele-
gant dinner hosted by a hospital foundation to honor a local physi-
cian's many years of service to the community. I accepted the writ-
ing assignment with only mild interest . . . at least until I placed
the first phone call to a colleague of the honoree.

"He's the finest doctor I've ever known," the fellow internist
reported simply. "He's the kind of role model every physician
could use."

A second call produced a comparable response: "His life gives
meaning to qualities like humanness, patience, and compassion,"
the family friend related. "He deals with humble people as if they
were important people and communicates sincerely with everyone
he touches. And he never limits himself in his relationships."

51

After several calls, I realized that the emerging portrait contained nothing about the man's clinical skills as a physician. While everyone with whom I spoke contributed some helpful and defining brushstroke, the observations and personal encounters had less to do with the doctor's professional achievements than with his character. But the award, as I understood it, was intended to honor his medical career. And, of course, it did. In fact, this man's career had opened him to a dimension of spirit that everyone recognized as healing.

Aside from his obvious kindness toward his patients, he seemed to inspire others in ways that helped them be well. His commitment to serve the life and people around him also strengthened the life within him and within his family. Though everyone insisted that he was a gifted physician, he had never let his professional training or clinical practice remove any aspects of wholeness from him. He had never allowed any conditions of the health care business world to erode his relationships or negatively alter his call to serve others through medicine.

Years earlier this physician had decided to let go of the typical clinical obsession with fascinating medical problems, and instead immersed himself in the daily routine of a healer. With compassion and awe, he attended to the souls of his patients as well as their bodies. He found that a patient's spirit was not just a human potential but a human need, and he learned that too much scientific objectivity can make a person blind to the whole picture of health and healing. Though his clinical skills rewarded him with a respected practice, he never lost sight of who he was and what he wished to share with the world. He seemed destined to care for others, to seek wholeness, and to recognize the value and dignity of each person he touched.

At the award ceremony, several eminent guests regaled the audience with glowing stories about the honored guest, showering him with well-deserved accolades. Finally, the time for presentations arrived, and the physician shyly approached the microphone *to make his acceptance speech. It was brief but, according to him, not brief enough.*

"There is nothing that becomes a person more than silence," he began. "Silence is a safeguard for wisdom." Thus, with a simple and gracious thank you, he returned to his seat. If anybody was disappointed at his lack of ceremony, they never showed it. Everyone seemed to understand perfectly.

In a place of quiet wisdom, this man had developed an uncanny ability to nourish and strengthen people. He practiced a rare kind of medicine: His listening ear and hospitable heart clearly informed his clinical competence. He embraced a simplicity synonymous with humility—a word derived from the Latin word humus, *earth. To be humble means to be in touch with the earth and all her inhabitants.*

We live in times of great uprootedness, when too little attention is paid to the wisdom of the heart. Some say that cardiac bypass surgery is a metaphor for our contemporary culture, a culture that has bypassed the heart. In many cases, alienation and cynicism have wounded us. Nagging doubts about the future of our careers and personal lives erode our self-confidence and optimism. From this queasy center emerges a fundamental truth— we need to connect with one another in sickness and health. We must sustain not just ourselves and our own dreams but also those of others and of the larger community. Our future hope and health rest in our capacity to reconsecrate our work and our personal lives. Whether we're healing professionals or simply trying to find the path toward wholeness, we all gain life when we realize that mystery sustains us much longer than does mastery.

Each of us is on a personal journey that offers limitless possibilities for healing encounters. Whether we teach school, care for children, or practice medicine, nobody and nothing can take away our choice of how we will respond to those encounters.

For instance, the physician faces a woman newly diagnosed with breast cancer. He steps down from his clinical pedestal, he removes the curtain that protects his heart, and he listens. A friend makes room in her busy day for another whose dreams have met head-on with limitation and failure. She touches the friend's hand and knows. An alcoholic finds freedom in recovery. He feels welcomed and challenged by his new AA family and wholesome friendships. A nurse places a cool cloth on the forehead of a fifteen-year-old girl who has just miscarried her baby. Sometimes a simple touch or gentle presence requires nothing more than silence to perform its healing work.

If the honored physician I've described brought a single priceless quality to his practice of medicine, it was the gift of attentive silence he offered each patient who walked through his office door. The fruit of this gift is a new possibility for a renewed humanity, one in which every woman and man can say yes to both self and others.

CHAPTER 10

Sometimes We Expect Too Much from Our Doctor

❧❧❧

Enlighten my mind that it may recognize what
   presents itself
And that it may comprehend what is absent or hidden.
Let it not fail to see what is visible
But do not permit it to arrogate to itself
The power to see what cannot be seen
For delicate and indefinite are the bounds
Of the great art of caring for the lives and health
   of your creatures.

—from "The Physician's Prayer,"
once attributed to Maimonides

A young woman named Jill described, in painful detail, her long ordeal with ulcerative colitis. This chronic inflammatory condition, characterized by tiny ulcers and small abscesses throughout the lining of the colon, had nearly destroyed her health. Not only had she lost a frightening amount of weight; she found it nearly impossible to eat even a small meal without suffering pain and the urgent need to move her bowels. Scared and despondent, Jill pressed on with her daily responsibilities, which included two jobs, and the care of her aging parents and her toddler.

Jill had done her homework well—at least her homework regarding her medical condition. She initiated an exhaustive literature search, visited several competent medical specialists, and made the rounds at an internationally acclaimed medical center. Unhappy with the answers and treatments she received from all the experts, she expanded her search into the field of complementary therapies. Jill tried acupuncture and spent time with a popular naturopath. She made appointments with massage therapists, herbalists, and a practitioner of traditional Chinese medicine. None offered her any relief; in fact, she became even more ill.

Finally, frustrated and angry with the entire medical establishment, Jill made an appointment at a local healing center whose comprehensive approach to treating illness included a variety of alternative therapies. Her first visit was supposed to include a thorough health history followed by a consultation with an internal medicine specialist who would coordinate her care. But by this time, Jill had no interest in holistic approaches to health. She was, in her words, tired of wasting precious time. Needless to say, the visit got off to a bad start and went further downhill when the center's dietitian recognized the need to involve other health professionals in her diagnosis and treatment plan. Jill stormed out and demanded a refund.

"I've done all that!" she exclaimed tearfully. "The last thing I need is for someone to take an inventory of the way I live. All I want is a diet that works."

Never during this whole process had Jill told her health practitioners that she was recently divorced. Nor did anybody learn about her struggles to balance child care with her professional perfectionism and her impossible work schedule. Her complicated, albeit productive life, "enhanced" by cellular phones and digital pagers, was literally squeezing the guts out of her.

Now she demanded a cure for an equally complicated medical condition.

Jill's expectations of the medical community seemed unrealistic, if not outright irrational. Yet the same could be said of society's expectations of Jill, and of Jill's expectations of herself. In fact, never did she seem to recognize or value her body's persistent protests against her lifestyle, nor did she see a need to attend to her self and soul. Lost somewhere in a vast array of prescription drugs and diagnostic procedures was Jill's assessment of what this illness meant to her. And it meant a lot. Colitis had become her life. Besides producing obvious physical pain, it left her feeling that she couldn't take care of herself anymore. Her productivity at work dropped dramatically, threatening her job security and causing her even more anxiety. In her search for a cure, Jill had ventured far outside her medical insurance coverage and had been left with huge bills. She lost health, money, clients, security, personal power, and autonomy.

No single element of Jill's situation held the answer to her health dilemma, but it's safe to say that she and countless women like her lead complex and depleting lives that defy health of body or soul. And expecting her physician to simply "fix" her was not realistic or fair. Yet to tell someone like Jill to simplify her life is not enough. She is the one who must discover what the life-giving asset called simplicity would mean to her.

If wisdom originates in simplicity, it also grows from simple daily events, from the plain encounters and unadorned stories that are ours. These are the windows through which we can rediscover the sense of certainty and the peace that inform good health. They also provide the foundations on which we can build our own formula for living well, something that Jill had never given a thought to.

AUTOIMMUNITY AND WOMEN

Autoimmunity, the underlying cause of over eighty serious
chronic illnesses, targets women approximately 75 percent
of the time. At a cost of some $86 billion a year, autoimmune
diseases occur when the immune system's method of recognizing foreign substances becomes confused. When this
occurs, the body manufactures immune cells called T-cells and
autoantibodies, which attack the body's own cells and organs.
These misguided T-cells and autoantibodies contribute to
many autoimmune diseases that implicate many medical spe-
cialties—rheumatology, endocrinology, neurology, cardiology,
gastroenterology, and dermatology. What launches the process that results in an autoimmune disease is not known.
While there has been little coordinated scientific attention to
the underlying causes of these diseases and why they are
more prevalent in women, research is looking at both the biological and psychosocial factors that might contribute to these
debilitating diseases.

While I was growing up, nobody warned me that my life
and the lives of many of my friends would be defined largely by
our ability to take care of ourselves and our children without a
spouse's help. Nor would I have guessed that mergers and management upsets would launch many of us from one job to
another, while we prayed to hang on to a paycheck, a little time
at the lake, and the possibility of working less someday. In the
world where I grew up, hardwood hillsides and rolling acres of
corn and alfalfa shaped the spiritual center from which I drew
nourishment. Today, I mine the essence of that time and place—
not in hopes of returning to the "good old days," but with a
kind of trust that says yes to the lessons of the earth that I
learned years ago.

Today, when I go home to visit, I again treasure the truth and rhythm of this quieter world, a place where, sometime late in August, summer stands still. This is when the season of planting and growing pauses to reflect before turning homeward toward autumn. The breeze drops to a sultry stillness. A subtle shift of air stretches the summer clouds across the humid sky. The piercing whir of cicadas punctuates the air in a place that waits for an abundant harvest. Corn has tasseled and oats are gone from the field. Round bales stand in tidy columns at the fence line. Grass along the roadside has gone to seed, and choke-cherries hang in heavy clusters from their spindly branches. It is a scene that says to me another growing season in the Midwest will drift quietly toward fruition. It is also a scene that calls me back to simpler truths.

This picture frames an average summer day in a world that now has little time for average. To be average is to fall short. Being average means not "doing" enough. A state of averageness veers dangerously close to failure. Being average doesn't pay es-pecially well, either. Instead, we hear that success comes through accomplishing above-average feats. Success means doing rather than being. We are what we do. We are important when we do something important. We are intelligent if we do something intelligent. We are valuable when we do something valuable. We are powerful if we do something powerful or, perhaps, when we take someone else's power away. This world, Jill's world, speaks little of health.

The problem with this world is that most of us, like the typ-ical August afternoon in the Wisconsin countryside, are pretty average. We experience almost the whole of our lives as com-mon days made up of small things and ordinary, oft-repeated transactions. The repetition of these events constitutes nearly our whole experience with one another and our world. I've come to believe that this kind of averageness points not to mediocrity, but to a divine energy, a greater reality that flows through the veins of our simple daily encounters. This kind of averageness can honestly inform our goals and values surrounding wholeness and health.

Excitement, ambition, and a thousand questionable causes may elevate us occasionally, but they will never replace the holiness of sharing a meal with a friend or holding the hand of someone who is anxious and alone. In the end, the real healing we experience comes not from what we acquire or achieve but from our willingness to be transformed—transformed as in the process of discovering the truth about ourselves and where we stand in relation to the world. By this process we take off the covers and reveal the light and success that are already there within us.

We are ultimately invited not just to attain but to set off on foot toward the August season, the season of our fruition. We are invited to walk on the holy ground of our human experience—the unspectacular and sometimes painful experience of becoming available to life and to one another. The true meaning of life, after all, lies hidden behind the ordinary. It speaks in quiet tones, not in high drama, but in the average. And sometimes, we begin to find health when we adjust our own course before looking outside to be fixed.

CHAPTER 11

Why Spirituality Matters

❧❦

*Religion and spirituality are "among the most important
factors that structure human experience, beliefs, values,
behavior and illness patterns."*

—Lukoff, *Journal of Nervous
and Mental Disease*

WHEN A PATIENT or family in the midst of a health crisis
starts asking me questions such as, "Why? How did this happen?" Or, "What does this mean?" I know that we are about to
have a conversation about God.

*A small circle of homeless men listened attentively as their coun-
selor announced the assignment. The faces might have belonged to
anyone anywhere. From professionals with postgraduate degrees
to the old and sickly, they came to the gospel mission from offices
and street corners, jails and reservations. They called themselves
late-stage, chronic alcoholics, and they were the men who huddle
beneath city bridges in the December cold sipping kerosene. Many
had gone again and again through local detox centers and shelters.
All were searching for a reason to hope.*

    *The counselor had asked them each to write a prayer. Every-
one managed to cobble together some words for the next meeting,
everyone except one older man. Each time the counselor asked how
he was coming along with the assignment, he simply shook his*

head. Years on the streets, immersed in alcohol and gloom, had left
him an empty vessel.

Week after week, the group met; the members of this recover-
ing community shared countless personal anecdotes. One week,
with the ragged group assembled once more, the counselor again
asked the man if he brought his prayer.

"Yes" was the reply, much to everyone's surprise. He then
pulled a crumpled bit of paper from his pocket and recited a
six-word entreaty: "Whoever made me, keep me safe."

The substance of this petition disclosed much about the person
who prayed it, and perhaps much about every one of us. It
revealed that at the core of every human being who has faced a
life-threatening crisis burns a soul searching for healing and for
connection with a source of strength and goodness beyond self.
Some would call this the spiritual search.

Spirituality is a popular concept, mentioned over and over
in today's self-help and complementary-medicine literature.
However, it still receives far too little attention from some health
professionals.

In modern medicine, spiritual language has been confined
to the recovery and religious communities, and this diminishes
the strength and fullness of its meaning. We often read about all
the things a person can do to improve his or her spiritual health,
but rarely do we hear about what it means to be a spiritually
whole person. In fact, even though spirituality lies at the heart
of AA's Twelve Steps and most world religions, misunderstanding of the term persists. For example, it's not often pointed out
that the Twelve Steps of AA simply provide one means of nurturing spiritual constructs such as simplicity, honesty, trust, and
humility—all basic, necessary ingredients of our human relationships and sense of well-being.

Each of us as a distinct and separate person possesses a
sense of isolation, of living within the boundaries of the self. Yet
we all also have a basic need to believe that we belong in the

world in some meaningful way. We inherently understand that we can transcend our separate selves. In part, the term "spirituality" is used to address this universal human longing for intimacy and community. To be spiritually complete implies that we understand our purpose in the world. To be spiritually whole means we have examined central issues of life, such as our understanding of ourselves and how we relate to others and the world we live in.

The spiritual dimension is difficult to define, let alone measure. It does not meet the objective criteria needed for scientific analysis. To some, its subjective manifestations may seem to involve wishful thinking, pathological projection, or the abandonment of rational analysis. Because of this, the spiritual dimension of health has not enjoyed a highly valued place in today's medical world.

The term "spirituality" is applied mainly to subjective phenomena. There are a number of concepts, however, that help to capture some elements of spirituality. The following encompass some (not all) of these elements, which can influence a person's health and capacity to cope with illness:

  A belief in some intrinsic meaning or order in the
      universe
  A faith that humanity and creation are inherently good
  An understanding that the force hidden in creation is a
      loving, present, and currently active energy
  A trust that this active energy behind creation could be
      called God or a Higher Power
  A willingness to accept what is; this is not to be confused
      with grudging resignation or with approval of evil
  A fundamental expectation of future good
  An ability to find peace of mind in an imperfect, ambiguous world
  A capacity to make peace with the knowledge that one's
      own personality is imperfect, although acceptable

Finally, growth or integration of one's inner or spiritual self ultimately produces a peaceful internal environment that nourishes flexibility, creativity, acceptance, trust, forgiveness, love, compassion, and hope.

"Spirit," derived from Latin, signifies breath or wind. It's basic to humankind, a vital element of our individual and collective humanity. Treatment professionals have long known that chemical dependency affects every part of a person, including that person's spirit. Thus, when someone begins to seek the fullness of living at a spiritual level, he also begins to recover from addiction.

A "spiritual awakening," according to treatment professionals, tends to help a person see and feel things he could not see or feel before. A spiritual awakening opens the door to knowledge previously hidden. This is how the Twelve Steps of Alcoholics Anonymous help people let go of their addictive selves and recognize their spiritual task of cultivating friendships and intimacy through simplicity, honesty, trust, and humility. It is at the level of spirit that one finds strength and identity through fellowship with others. This is the place where power comes from something larger than self, a source of wisdom that can guide us as we grow and change.

Spirituality defined in these terms encompasses a spirituality of movement toward completion or wholeness. It accentuates companionship—friend with friend, helping, sharing, celebrating, and even despairing. The spiritual essence moves us toward a relationship with the universe, with others, and with our self. It asks, "Who am I? Where do I find meaning and purpose in life? How do I bond with others?"

A spirituality of wholeness invites the deepest forms of human healing. This healing lives in our present and daily experience of one another. It says, "I will help someone for no other reason than that she needs help. I will live out a life of compassion as a vital act of creation. I will make justice by acting mercifully." This spirituality offers free and cordial emptiness for others to enter—offers a space where souls can get acquainted. It shatters our illusions of having it all together, of having control or of attaining personal perfection. It reminds us that we are called not to do big things but to do small things well. Finally, it challenges us to walk with hope on an uncharted footpath called life.

A spirituality of wholeness speaks of simplicity. To be humble means to be in touch with the earth and all who inhabit it, to be reconciled and made whole. The humble host knows that each guest carries precious gifts. This spirituality says that, upon discovering our unique nature, we also find that we are one with the homeless man. His prayer could be our prayer.

"Whoever made me, keep me safe."

This is ultimately a prayer of belief, a belief that we are indeed part of a sweeping plan that includes much more than our own dilemma and our own space. This kind of trust says that we can search our hearts, make amends, be reconciled, and hope for reconciliation whenever we choose.

CHAPTER 12

Learn to Trust the Power of Plain and Small Things

❧❧

God, kindle thou in my heart within
a flame of love to my neighbor,
to my foe, to my friend,
to my kindred all,
to the brave, to the knave, to the thrall,
of Son of the loveliest Mary,
from the lowliest thing that liveth
to the name that is highest of all.

—A Celtic prayer

YOU COULD CALL IT *nature's last hurrah for the year. Certainly October, with its bright skies and brilliant color, provides one of my native Wisconsin's finest selling points. Yet, along with its beauty, a sense of the tragic surrounds this mysterious month. The leaves reach the height of glory just before they flutter to the ground to die. The earth, having given up its harvest of grain, suddenly turns inward to rest. In October we see the coming and going of life.*

October raises questions about human potential and human limitations. On one hand, it washes the countryside with exquisite pigments. On the other hand, it reminds us that we will soon face winter and its challenges and hardships. October also exposes the fragile nature of all life, including human life. This is the month

67

of Halloween, or Samhain, a Celtic word meaning summer's end. According to ancient tradition, this celebration of Samhain marked the beginning of the season of hope and of memory, when the gods came and walked upon the earth for a while. And according to pre-Christian religious traditions in Britain and Ireland, October marked the beginning of the sacred season during which the earth and her inhabitants retreated to their roots to be rejuvenated.

In October we should look beyond the brief cycles of nature and her killing frosts toward meaningful truths that hold up through the years. The October mystery encourages us to ask ourselves, "How is it we choose to lead our lives? How do we maintain faith and confidence in a world of such turbulence? How do we live well? Where can we turn for sustenance and goodness?"

The Jewish theologian Abraham Heschel says that the spiritual life is a matter not of acquiring information but of learning to see the world in a new way. Sometimes it might even be a matter of learning to see the world in an old way. Unfortunately, contemporary American culture does not yet show much interest in this approach of feeling, listening, and intuitively sensing the world's wisdom. We complicate faith with intellectual and doctrinal standards, while we complicate the rest of our lives with clutter. No wonder one of Alcoholics Anonymous's most popular suggestions for keeping spiritually well is "Keep it simple."

We chaplains who work with children learn early on that keeping it simple means everything to the people we meet. Their lives have already become enormously complicated. Rarely do we get to visit or play with well children. Mostly we find parents already exhausted, keeping vigil in a surgery waiting room, an intensive care unit, or a newborn intensive care nursery. In these settings, families must give away much of their power. Like it or not, they have to let go of the selves that can supervise things, organize things, and control things—even things as simple as daily schedules and privacy. While hospital caregivers march confidently through their medical task lists, families find themselves having to trust and wait. Parents feel exceedingly vulnerable and often bond with other families in similar circumstances. As the minutes and hours pass, social barriers dissolve. Complete strangers cling together, held by a tender thread of hope mixed with a large dose of apprehension.

Most of us experience hospitals as places where complicated, even heroic, acts take place—especially a hospital exclusively for children where sophisticated technology can save the life of a baby born at twenty-four weeks' gestation. Surgeons perform intricate heart procedures on down-covered infants who fit neatly in the palm of an adult hand. Other medical specialists operate complicated ventilators that sustain the lives of tiny babies whose lungs have not yet developed. I have witnessed spectacular medical miracles at the hands of astute neonatologists and pediatric neurosurgeons.

Yet, in spite of these lifesaving deeds, I'm often captivated by how the extraordinary breaks into ordinary daily events, even in a hospital. Feeding, bathing, housekeeping, teaching, and praying—these are the routine elements of care that take on new meaning for the people living in this world. Far more than kind acts of concern, they become powerful signs of continuity. Somehow these basic tasks, performed day by day and year by year, generate a rhythmic and life-sustaining cycle that truly can be trusted. I view it as certain proof that the "center" still holds!

The Celtic approach to God opens up a world where nothing is too common to be exalted and nothing is so exalted that it cannot be made common. Heaven lies "a foot and a half above the height of man," said an old woman from Kerry, in the southwest of Ireland. The Celts have provided the world with a wealth of prayers and poems from the frontiers of England, Wales, Scotland, and Ireland. Celtic spirituality, once almost forgotten, has enjoyed a strong revival during the past decade. Its humble, homely approach to God was born out of harsh lives, often spent in conditions of extreme poverty and relentless work.

The Celts were ordinary people who took the tasks of their daily lives and treated them sacramentally. Celtic spirituality took common things and interpreted them as signs of a greater reality. Getting up in the morning and carrying out one's tasks of washing, making the fire, milking and weaving, fishing and farming testified to a holy presence in creation. Nearly everything that happened between birth and death could become an occasion for recognizing the closeness of God.

Viewed in its entirety, the Celtic approach to spiritual life offers both reassurance and honesty. Too often, the religious or spiritual messages we receive say that God's presence can only be confirmed in certain places or through prescribed events, by some revolutionary improvement or radical conversion. Likewise, secular human successes come only through the highest level of achievement. Rarely is anyone rewarded for being somewhere in the middle, and certainly not for being plain or modest. Servanthood and humility do not rate highly on the American priority list. The problem with this is that most of us don't find our days filled with newsmaking acts, front-page deeds, or headline tributes.

How easy it is to fall into the trap of believing that any hope of attaining the good life lies in our ability to earn our way in through our accomplishments. Our space might feel more hospitable if we learned to simply live out each day in the knowledge that success is as close as our simple routines and small commitments. It's those shared, ordinary events and stale transactions that keep us grounded and well. They make up the loom on which we weave a strong and serviceable garment. This idea might be one of the most profound though difficult truths that we ever learn.

Each of us is ultimately called not to achieve or attain but to make his or her own path toward peace. We are invited to walk on the sacred ground of our human experience, the ordinary, unspectacular, and sometimes painful experience of our time together. Each day furnishes us with new adventures and new paths toward completion. Each passing year shines new light on the meaning of our days.

Whether we speak of Celtic spirituality, routines at work and at home, or the predictable patterns of a hospital community, we benefit by attending to plain things. What we really need is to celebrate life together. What we really long for is to be together in community and simply enjoy the beauty of creation. Yet we often let a mountain of obstacles prevent us from being where our hearts want to be. We get caught up in the battle for survival, the hectic, pressured, competitive, exhausting experience of life. We must remember the gift that waits to be accepted—the gift that lives in all the homely circumstances of each day.

LISTENING   *To listen: to hear, attend closely to, heed, give ear, and give audience. To listen requires silencing ourselves so as to create an empty space in which another person can feel safe expressing his or her ideas, needs, and fears. Listening lies at the heart of medicine. It also lies at the heart of justice, love, and peace. Our need to listen is surpassed only by our need to connect with one another on a deep level of human experience.*

CHAPTER 13

Return to Your Senses

*Should all the saints and angels of heaven join with all the
members of the church on earth, both religious and lay at
every degree of Christian holiness and pray for my growth
in humility, I am certain it would not profit me as much nor
bring me to perfection of this virtue as quickly as a little
self-knowledge.*

—Unknown fourteenth-century English mystic,
The Cloud of Unknowing

THE POET ROBERT FROST often wrote of the seasons; in his
poem "November," he described the subtle beauty of late fall.
The poem also captures the mood of the quiet interlude before
winter, a reflective time when we start to prepare for months of
cold and ice. November, for those of us who live in the Midwest,
is nature's shroud donned in preparation for an icy assault.

Each of our seasons speaks from its own mystery. Each
reveals messages about life's passages and the inner flow of time.
In late October and November, the mood of fall changes; leaving
their brilliant colors, the days take on the more subtle shades of
quiet mornings and early darkness. The end of daylight saving
time directs us toward inward thoughts. Though November signals the dying of a year, it does not mean the dying of hope or
the end of growth. November marks both the death of summer
and the start of life's temporary retreat, a turn back to its roots in

search of new energy. November is about becoming recharged for the next leg of the journey. In fact, a look at my neighbors' garden reveals that horse chestnut trees and maples had already set their buds for spring.

With this in mind, one Thanksgiving dawn I pulled on warm clothes and set out for an early walk. We lived in a neighborhood of lovely Victorian homes strung along quiet brick streets. Giant white oaks stood guard along the boulevards, their leaves still clinging to the branches, braced against a sky that told of a coming snowfall. Gray squirrels scampered through the dry leaves to rush up the half-naked English ivy climbing on the stately homes. Highbush cranberries and naked lilac bushes framed an austere city skyline.

Strolling through the leaves and deserted culs-de-sac, I observed the first glimmers of lamplight deep within the handsome dwellings. The neighborhood slowly began to awaken. Watching households emerge from inky darkness filled me with a sensation of closeness to all those who stirred inside. I imagined them shuffling about in their bathrobes or sitting at the kitchen table with a hot cup of coffee. Some probably prayed, or worried, or simply read the morning newspaper. Within hours their houses would overflow with the commotion of family and holiday guests. It all served as a quiet reminder that there is life after November.

We are, in some ways, products of our earth's seasons. The fall calls us to reach into the depths of our lives, to examine our courses and perhaps redirect them. We move indoors and enter the interior recesses of our hearts. In both cases, the watchwords are "wait" and "listen." Wait for snow. Wait for cold. Wait for spring. Wait and search for wisdom.

Meanwhile, we do our waiting in a world that persists in doing and accomplishing much more than it considers the implications of its actions. The computer programmer has become the scribe of our society, recording at warp speed our deeds and discoveries. René Descartes, a sixteenth-century French philosopher, often receives credit for creating our present world-view. It is a philosophical system that has fostered the tremendous growth of both science and education. Cartesian thought combined with the introduction of the printing press brought the spread of ideas and literature throughout Europe. With the establishment of this way of observing the world, knowledge became information *about* things and people rather than a personal encounter with life. Knowledge was gathered and recorded, a fact at a time. The long journey from printed words to bits of data, the word processor, and then the computer had begun.

Before all this, we lived in a sensuous world, a world in which people relied on the ear and all the sense organs. Reality was experienced by sight, hearing, touch, smell, and taste. The oral story held a position of great importance to cultural health and history. A November walk into darkness could be trusted to reveal enduring truths. Obviously none of our senses disappeared with the introduction of science and technology, but today, the world about which they tell us has become suspect. If we can't come up with hard evidence that something exists, not many people are ready to believe it. The soulful experience remains dubious and lacking in credibility. In such a world, personal reflection and prayerful conviction risk being seen as time-wasting obstacles rather than as trustworthy sources of truth. We learn that what we know is more important then how we care. We worship competency and believe we must always be doing something that produces results. In such a world we have become ashamed of the heart and of all implications of softness.

Some say New Age spirituality and today's popular quest to recover ancient healing traditions are reactions to Descartes's world. Many of these traditions attempt to recover some of the priceless acoustical senses amidst our encounters with life. Mainstream medicine is also making an effort to think more holistically. This is important because, despite its value, Descartes's worldview defines life merely as what is material and observable. It defines life on very stingy terms.

So, in the month when the earth and her inhabitants settle into violet stillness, perhaps it's life itself that waits for us to return to our senses. One can only hope so.

CHAPTER 14

Nourishing the Body Can Heal the Soul

❦

A Kitchen Blessing

Give us, O god our morning meal
your gift for the body
and food for the soul.
Encompass this kitchen;
inspire its cooks
with joy of preparing
and serving
and sharing.

A WOMAN SPOKE *of her son, who had come home to live with her after a ten-year absence. A magnificent athlete and promising musician, this gifted young man had abandoned college only to tumble headlong into a mire of drugs and despair. His family and friends watched, powerless, as he continued his free fall toward a terrifying abyss.*

His mother struggled to describe a torturous decade of the boy's misadventures—drunk driving arrests, motorcycle wrecks, ruined friendships, lost employment, late-night phone calls, threatened suicide, and multiple attempts to get medical help. Creditors' letters arrived, demanding delinquent payments. Complete strangers called to express concern for his safety. Family and friends held their collective breath, suspended in dread. Many tried to intervene. Many more gave in or gave up. The boy rejected every invitation to reclaim his life. Instead, he careened dangerously into deeper darkness.

Finally, one day, for no clear reason, the young man simply came home. Perhaps he knew something better awaited him there. Maybe he grasped, ever so dimly, the consequences of traveling further down the path he had chosen for himself. More than likely, he just ran out of money and places to hide. The reason for his return hardly mattered to his mother. He simply showed up at the kitchen door one morning.

His blank gaze startled his mother. Everything about him seemed out of sync and out of touch. She felt strangely uneasy sitting close to him, being alone in the house with him. Pale and empty, he displayed not a hint of the child she had raised. Where had he been all this time? Who had he become? How might she care for him and help restore him to some semblance of health? Was there any hope of mending such a damaged vessel? Finally, how could the two of them hope to find success together now, as an enforced community of two?

They sat together in relative silence, she maneuvering gingerly around the missing years. Time suspended. Time gone. A virtual stranger was looking back at her from across the kitchen table. Her thoughts whirled. All she knew about addiction and "Toughlove" seemed hopelessly unsuitable for this situation. She groped for a sign or some helpful insight. The counselors had never told her what was supposed to happen next. She waited in clumsy silence for some profound piece of wisdom to surface. Nothing did. At last, guided only by intuition, she got up from her chair, kissed her son, and went to the kitchen stove to prepare him a meal. For the next year, she quite literally fed him back to health.

Food wields a mighty power. It provides comfort to heart, body, and soul. Food is a universal language; it connects one to another even when other familiar avenues of connection have closed.

The day this mother began cooking with love for her wounded son, she somehow infused that love into her meals. By preparing food and breaking bread with him for many months, she offered him a sustaining energy and power of life. Sharing the gift of food implicated her in her son's struggle for life. It brought her into community with him and created an intimacy that might never have been achieved otherwise. The food she provided nourished both his body and his soul. In the midst of confusion and doubt she intuitively created a nourishing environment in which he could begin to recover his health and personhood.

In studying the food-related beliefs of various wisdom traditions, the nutritionist Deborah Kesten discovered that honoring food through thoughtful preparation, then partaking of it with depth and sincerity, actually makes it sacred. Food is sanctified by warmth and affection. She found that many traditions offer a spiritual perspective that we have forgotten over the centuries: When we furnish food with such sacred understanding, it will nourish both body and soul. When we partake of food in this manner, we also contribute in an essential way to healing.

Most cultures and religions have rituals that use food as a means of connecting to a deeper spiritual significance. Jewish dietary laws, for example, honor the sanctity of the life inherent in both animal- and plant-based food. Christians sustain their connection to Jesus Christ through the bread and wine of Holy Communion. African Americans season their soul food with love as a way of celebrating community and friendships. Yogis eat, in part, to commune with food's life-giving qualities, while Muslims honor food for its divine essence. Buddhists pursue enlightenment by bringing a meditative awareness to food. The Chinese communicate with the gods through food, and the Japanese turn to tea to renew the spirit.[1]

While food as spiritual sustenance enjoys a long and rich history in countless cultures, traditional nutritional science, much like traditional Western medicine, has been based primarily on biology. Nutritional science attempts to understand, explain, or control the content of our food, and in this way it provides an incomplete picture based on a particular worldview.

The view of food as no more than a collection of nutrients springs from the same scientific method that has shaped today's biomedical model of medicine. The scientific developments of the seventeenth century—including the mathematical formulas by which Isaac Newton predicted the movement of the planets—inspired the same mechanistic approach to food as to medicine. These developments ultimately found Western civilization looking at life—including the human body—as a machine that could be measured, fixed, and fueled.

Ultimately, nutritional scientists learned to break down foods into proteins, fats, carbohydrates, and minerals. The calorie, a measure of food energy established by the French chemist Antoine Laurent Lavoisier in the eighteenth century, added to the measurement tools.

The popular media today demonstrate how our view of diet and nutrition continues to reflect this mechanistic approach. Diet and health publications remain preoccupied with marking and measuring the contents of food. Our focus on calories, fat content, and how cooking and processing change the nutrient value of food reveals that we still treat food as the fuel that runs or clogs the human engine. Vitamins, minerals, and all manner of other food supplements have become popular, albeit expensive, tools to drive the body and tune up human physical and intellectual performance. Even today's seemingly more balanced approach to nutrition breaks the body down into separate

parts—heart, brain, or colon—with each part requiring a specific nutritional fix. While nobody would deny the value of research related to fat, sugar, and calories in our diet, excessive
focus on nutrition can take away from the sensual pleasure and
enjoyment of eating.

But the spiritual potential of food encompasses everything
from the soil that produces what we eat, to the thoughtful act of
preparing and sharing meals. Food, in a most profound way,
brings us into community with others to listen, smell, and taste.
Food tends to encourage intimacy and foster feelings of safety
and well-being. Food often sparks memories. It naturally invites
storytelling.

All of this probably explains why my mother always kept a
food journal. Nowhere in its pages could we find any notations
about how many calories or grams of sugar were in her graham
cracker cake or her crown roast of pork. Instead, she filled every
line with lists of friends who had come for Christmas dinner.
She included the size of the turkey or roast beef she served,
noted what people wore to Christmas dinner, and jotted recipes
for open-face sandwiches to be served at tea. She noted snippets
of cooking instructions, commented on her favorite dishes,
made timetables, and listed birthday cake choices. Food for her
clearly delivered more than nourishment to her guests. She
understood its power and she used it in a most hospitable way.

The young man who came home from his misadventure also
benefited from the healing qualities of food. Whether he immediately recognized it or not, he soon began to understand that
all of life was interconnected through the process of food preparation. The connection exists through the soil and rain, the
workers who cultivate and harvest food, and the cook who prepares it. All are joined in a most profound and potentially healing way.

He also began to benefit from the familiar routines surrounding food preparation and sharing. He grew to appreciate

the predictability of sitting down together with others, the safety and comfort of predictable rituals. As his energy grew, so did his hope. Eating with others who cared about him became a point of celebration and brightness. Slowly, over the course of time, he reacquainted himself with the textures and flavors of food and with the community of family who wished him good health. His homecoming ultimately became a cause for celebration.

Usually, when we talk about celebration, we mean festive events such as holidays, reunions, and anniversaries. We remember times when we have been able to forget the burdens of life and immerse ourselves in an atmosphere of music and merriment for a while. But celebration in a spiritual sense is more than a party. This kind of celebration occurs only through the deep realization that life and death are never found completely separate. It can come about only when fear and love, joy and sorrow, weeping and laughter, birth and death can coexist without overwhelming us. Hence, to break bread with another human being is to celebrate by sharing the sustaining energy and power of life.

GRANDMA COOK'S CELEBRATION CAKE

In its celebratory tradition, our family, like many others, enjoyed a favorite cake, which appeared at birthday parties, picnics, and whenever we felt an occasion deserved some kind of observation. This cake breaks most nutritional rules, and it tastes divine.

2 cups sugar
1 cup unsalted butter, room temperature
3 large eggs
1 cup graham cracker crumbs, crushed fine with a rolling pin
1 cup milk
1 cup chopped walnuts
1 cup shredded sweetened coconut

1$^3/_4$ cups white flour, sifted before measuring
2 teaspoons baking powder
1 tablespoon vanilla

PREHEAT oven to 350 degrees and set oven racks in the middle. Cream butter and sugar together to a light, rich cream. Add eggs one at a time, beating well between each addition. Blend flour and baking powder and add alternately with milk. Add vanilla. Fold in coconut and chopped walnuts.

GREASE and flour three 8-inch round baking pans. Divide batter among pans and bake until toothpick tests done. Cool slightly before removing cakes from pans to cool completely.

Filling:
1 pint heavy cream, whipped
$^1/_2$ cup sugar
2 teaspoons vanilla
2 cups fresh pineapple chunks
2 large bananas, sliced
1 pint basket raspberries or strawberries

WHIP cream to soft peaks and add vanilla and sugar. Continue whipping until consistency is good for spreading. Place first cake layer on a large plate and cover with whipped cream. Cover the cream with $^1/_3$ of the fruit. Place second cake on top of first and repeat the process. Add third layer, fruit, and whipping cream. Cover sides of cake and decorate top with reserved berries. Celebrate!

CHAPTER 15

Why It's Important to Make Time for Community

※❦※

To SAY THAT community fosters health is to say that July can get humid in Minnesota—an outlandish understatement. Over and over I have seen through the eyes of patients and colleagues that community provides an essential ingredient in preserving and restoring health. Thus, the rare group of chaplains with whom I have worked concluded early on that, if we truly valued the therapeutic benefits of community, we had better make a genuine attempt to live it.

Through the years, our faithful assemblage has looked more like an affirmative action poster than a spiritually mature group of religious professionals. We make up a curious stew of cultures, colors, ages, religious traditions, and communication styles. Singularly overqualified and often overworked, most of us fulfill several other professional assignments outside the hospital. We have been called opinionated and silly. We also have been known to err, occasionally, on the side of irreverence. This, too, is therapeutic.

Like everyone else we know, all of us wrestle with overfull calendars. Lost time cards, forgotten call schedules, and sometimes mismatched methods of conflict resolution color our canvas, as well. Fortunately, we all like our work and one another—fortunately, because the vocation we choose to follow is not one intended for sissies.

A quick assessment of our spiritual care team reveals a host of potential obstacles that could stand in the way of closeness. We are five startlingly unalike individuals—five clear reasons why many people cling to those who look like them and think as they do. How much simpler and more efficient work would be if we were five middle-aged Episcopalian women clergy (simpler for me, that is). Instead, our many differences mean we must listen more carefully, negotiate more fully, and build plans more thoughtfully. Doing so might require more work, but we all have appreciated the rewards.

So, with an eye on silliness and a commitment to our success together, we work hard at maintaining our somewhat eccentric little community. We talk often, sharing personal and professional wins and losses. We hang out together as much as is reasonable. At least once a month, we spend the evening together, away from the hospital. We do not use this time to discuss quality improvement or budgets. These get-togethers consist of serious recreation as well as heartfelt discussions. Sometimes our families come, and sometimes we come alone. It matters little who or how many appear at the door. Sometimes curious newcomers join us and have so much fun they decide to join us again . . . permanently. Our boss (who is not a chaplain) comes. So does a neighborhood priest who has grown tired of spending supper hour rattling around in his empty rectory. Showing up is the important thing, and our evenings have proven to be a wonderfully potent prescription for the isolation and exhaustion that cling to a soul hours after the daily drill has drawn to a close.

This place where we meet speaks of hospitality. Hospitality not only informs our community (and all communities), but has also enjoyed a long relationship with the original concept of a hospital. Established by early monastic communities and often connected with churches and cathedrals, hospitals served as havens for weary travelers, welcoming oases offering food and rest to anyone who needed either. Even today, one can find hospitals, such as those in Pisa and Siena, Italy, that are designed to care for the poor and tired sojourner as well as for the sick and elderly.

Hospitality, then, anticipates the arrival of guests. It requires a welcoming heart that knows and accepts our own and another's incompleteness. To offer hospitality within community is to weave together a common cloth of gladness and defeat, of shared routines and daily plans. With mighty fibers secured as one, hospitality impels us to become whole.

Why Community Is Necessary

We live in a time when considerable value has been attached to rugged individualism. Don't cry. Don't risk revealing your authentic self. Win often. Crave much. Do well. Attain more. Wear the macho mask—or whatever mask disguises you most completely. This kind of individualism crushes the heart and energy of community. It can also crush the vitality of our bodies and spirits.

Community, though often associated with religious institutions, exists within any intimate group. A community can be little or big, biologically related or professionally connected. In sickness and in health, community furnishes the mortar that binds up human brokenness and restores hope. A community consists of individuals who choose to be together so that they might communicate deeply and honestly with one another. Community meets people where they are—rejoicing, sharing

---

REENERGIZING RELATIONSHIPS

Strong relationships with supportive friends, helpmates, and colleagues provide a foundation on which we thrive. These relationships affect everything from our understanding of truth to our level of self-esteem, from our motivation to engage in life to our commitment to caring for ourselves. While it is easy to take close relationships for granted, it is essential to feed those relationships in order to keep them strong and well. The following recommendations can add new life to important relationships.

• Express sincere appreciation to another person. Remind that person of how much she or he means to you. Focus on individual strengths and offer genuine, regular compliments. Acknowledge this person's positive contributions to your day.
• Set dates to spend time in the company of people whose relationships you value. Choose something new to do together. Pack a lunch to share. Review your calendar regularly, making certain you keep appointments with those people who hold a place of prominence in your life.

---

frustrations, or mourning losses. It asserts that individuality and interdependence are not mutually exclusive. It calls us to become fully ourselves while remaining joined to another or others. Community nourishes children while it sustains adults and protects fragile elders.

Difficult as it sometimes seems, we must try to make time to come together simply to enjoy one another. Refreshment lies in celebrating life together simply—sharing good food, teasing, laughing, and restoring selves depleted by our daily responsibilities. It might seem a small and unnecessary thing, but it helps.

- Communicate often with those close to you. Find times to connect, and set those times aside from the daily routines. Whether you send an e-mail message or a card, or take a coffee break together, use your time to listen and to speak of things that matter to both of you.

- Consider ways of strengthening your spiritual lives individually and together. Enter into spiritual or cultural activities within and beyond your faith traditions. Identify what nourishes you spiritually (meditation, gardening, painting, keeping a journal), and make time for it.

- Make your relationships a high priority. Despite busy schedules, investing time and energy in relationships is absolutely imperative. Listen to and learn to recognize another's needs. Assure that person that you care about her or his well-being and plan to be there during times of difficulty as well as times of fun.

- Learn to reframe conflicts in your relationships as windows of opportunity. Seek help from trusted friends or professionals. Explore other resources to help nurture your relationships and move you through challenging times.

CHAPLAINS' CHICKEN

Our small community of chaplains has represented so many cultures and tastes, one might have thought it difficult to settle on a food that everyone enjoyed. But we did. Chicken always seems to work, and the following recipe, adapted to suit all of us, has been a winner . . . hence the name, chaplains' chicken.

1 cup chopped fresh parsley

1 cup chopped fresh basil

1 cup grated Parmesan cheese

$^3/_4$ cup chopped pecans
3 cloves garlic
$^1/_4$ cup vermouth or other dry white wine
$^1/_2$ cup buttermilk
$^1/_3$ cup peanut oil
6 skinned chicken breasts
Pinch of cayenne pepper

PREHEAT oven to 350 degrees.

COMBINE parsley, Parmesan cheese, basil, and pecans. Reserve one cup of this mixture for sprinkling on top of chicken.

BLEND remaining parsley mixture, garlic, vermouth, and buttermilk in a blender or food processor until smooth.

TURN blender or processor on high and gradually add oil in a slow, steady stream.

ARRANGE chicken breasts in an ungreased baking dish and add salt and pepper to taste. Pour blended parsley-vermouth-buttermilk mixture over chicken; sprinkle with reserved cup of parsley mixture.

BAKE at 350 degrees for one hour.

COMPASSION   *To be compassionate is to assume a posture of heartfelt tenderness, benevolence, mercy, favor, thoughtfulness, gentleness, caring, and responsiveness toward self and others. To act compassionately is to enter into the human suffering of another and share that person's burden of sickness or sorrow. Compassion guides the way from human brokenness to wholeness.*

CHAPTER 16

The Courage to Cope
with Chronic Illness

❧❦

The soul grows by subtraction, not by addition.
                    —Meister Eckhart

*For at least the past generation, our society has roman-
ticized and revered standards of health and fitness to the
exclusion of the less healthy and the less fit. Unfortunately,
the reality of chronic illness has been neglected.*

                    —Howard Steven Shapiro, M.D.

D R . SHAPIRO'S MESSAGE *has never made it into the ad copy
for any popular running shoe. Nor does it grace the pages of high-
fashion magazines. In fact, advertisements continue to offer the
sunny notion that diet, exercise, nutrition, and cosmetics can solve
virtually anyone's beauty and health problems. In 1987, it was estimated that some 90 million Americans were living with a chronic
condition; 39 million of those were living with more than one.
Over 45 percent of noninstitutionalized Americans reported one
or more chronic conditions, and their direct health care costs
accounted for three-fourths of U.S. health care expenditures.
Total costs projected to 1990 for people with chronic conditions
amounted to $659 billion—$425 billion for direct health care costs
and $234 billion in indirect costs.*[1]

A woman named Eleanor thinks the consumer message of "easy" health stinks. A mother, homemaker, author, and patient advocate, Eleanor speaks with authority when she says the prevalence and costs of chronic conditions as a whole have rarely been estimated. Eleanor has lived with systemic lupus erythematosus for the past dozen years. She also knows what it feels like to grow up in a society that believes suffering is akin to a social accident and can be avoided by making good investments, working hard, and taking care of yourself. She now knows a different reality, and the emotional price of that truth was high.

Lupus, from the Latin for wolf, gets its name from an accompanying skin condition that resembles a wolf bite. Systemic lupus is a chronic inflammatory disease that may affect the skin, joints, kidneys, and central nervous system. It is commonly characterized by periods of remission and relapse; complications sometimes arise from its treatment with high doses of corticosteroids or immunosuppressive drugs.

"It didn't take me long to realize that I was not going to be one of the exceptional few to recover from a chronic illness," said Eleanor. The first six months after her diagnosis were bad times for her and her family as they battled with what she admits were overwhelming emotional and physical changes. Eleanor spent more than four of those six months hospitalized with symptoms ranging from difficulty breathing to unexplained fevers. She found herself teetering on the brink of emotional collapse, yet she also recognized the dangers of languishing within her illness.

"I don't know whether I became well enough or things just evolved that way, or how exactly it happened, but I made a decision that I was going to find out all that I could find out about my disease and then share that information with others." At that point, Eleanor not only moved beyond her immediate medical and personal crisis but also began to function as an advocate for anyone and everyone challenged by chronic illness.

At that time, the Internet was relatively undeveloped and was not widely used. Eleanor quickly ascertained that most libraries held precious little current information on chronic disease. For example, through her own research, she was shocked to find a fifteen-year-old statistic that claimed lupus was terminal to all but 10 percent of those who contracted it. "I realized if I was getting that kind of health information, then everyone else was, too," she said. "However, I had a fundamental intellectual curiosity and interest in things. That kept me going."

Eleanor then got down to ferreting out correct, pertinent, and timely data, first through support groups, local disease associations, and computerized library searches. Then she began sharing her information with support group members. Others prodded her to write a book on chronic illness, and eventually her compromised health placed Eleanor on the path to an unexpected career.

Meanwhile, a friend of hers, a woman named Allie, was facing each day armed with her own steady stream of drugs and devices. One medical professional called her condition chronic obstructive lung disease. Another saw a pattern of acute and chronic asthma. To Allie, it mattered little what name the medical professionals gave her problem. Her vocabulary consisted of words like "bronchodilator," "nebulizer," "theophylline," and "corticosteroid." Every day meant a rigid schedule of therapy for a mixed bag of illness that literally took her breath away.

The trouble with lung patients, according to Allie's respiratory therapists, is they never get well, although they experience better times and worse times. Allie, however, never knew times when she could breathe easily. Her treatment was both complex and time consuming: complex, because she was trying to maintain a delicate balance of powerful medicines while avoiding their side effects; time-consuming, because her therapy required four one-hour breathing treatments a day—without fail.

Allie's health had started to deteriorate after she underwent surgery for a back injury she received at work. After convalescing for several weeks, she tried unsuccessfully to return to her job. But her coughing and bouts of asthma became so persistent that even less strenuous jobs such as telemarketing were out of the question. After twenty-five years, Allie's career as a supervisor in a large manufacturing company had come to an end. Nagging questions about her future health and livelihood began to surface. She had always thought that every problem, including health problems, had a solution. If you felt sick, you called in a prescription. If you broke a bone, you fixed it. According to this system, she had been cheated.

Yet Allie refused to cave in to health restrictions. Instead of succumbing to the obvious pitfalls of depression and despair, she reshaped her life into a productive and remarkably active regime. Not that she has escaped the dark side of chronic illness; she has even thought about some pretty bleak options.

"It sometimes feels like I have five dollars in the bank and I just spent ten," she explained. "But if I take my own life, I've taken a precious gift. I have finally made peace with myself."

Most of us know an Eleanor or an Allie. Most of us have witnessed someone living out a life of dubious quality and wondered where she or he came upon such a tenacious spirit. They somehow find an inner strength that refuses to be crushed by disheartening losses, debilitating disease, and misfortune that could be expected to stagger the most robust person. These are the ones who adjust. They keep marching on—not with a "There's a lesson in this for me" attitude, but with a simple expectancy that something worthwhile waits on the next horizon. They are the ones who learn to walk through the furnace of pain without being consumed by it.

One of the most striking characteristics of the Eleanors and Allies of this world is their ability to let go and open themselves. Maybe one learns this when situations become unmanageable, or maybe the ability to let go was an aspect of each woman's character before she became chronically ill. In either case, both women made major adjustments in their lives, continuing to recenter themselves in response to their constantly changing conditions.

"Some days I hate my body," said Eleanor, "but I refuse to let it capture me. When you have a chronic condition, you sometimes need to disconnect from your body and disregard some of your symptoms or you couldn't do anything."

Both women found they could let go of their past—not just their previous good health, but their past physical activities, goals, aspirations, guilt, and even some past relationships. Not that they threw up their hands; they took inventory of their resources and limitations and concluded that certain things had to go. Tedious meetings and daily jogging were out. Adaptive exercise equipment and simple suppers were in.

One does not have to be chronically ill to see the value of letting go. Each of us who has set out on a search for fulfillment has probably already encountered the disappointment, frustration, and resentment that spill over us when plans are wrecked. Sometimes we set such a hard-and-fast framework of conditions for ourselves that we become easy prey to disillusionment. And disappointment persists when we can't bring ourselves to loosen our grip on the shape of our plans.

By placing rigid restrictions on our course and insisting that we stage all our scenes, we set ourselves up for immeasurable disappointment. But when we agree to turn our lives over, in some degree, to a creative energy, we learn to trust the direction in which life steers us. Some specific qualities can actually help this process.

Knowing our own value rates among the most essential of these qualities. Too often, people confuse genuine self-love or caring for self with selfishness and egotism. Actually, egocentricity indicates a morbid preoccupation with self and a blindness to the needs of others. Truly selfish people have trouble loving others, and they seldom love themselves.

IDEAS FOR LIVING WITH CHRONIC ILLNESS

The continuing debates about health care reform remind us of what a high value we place on health and longevity. How long we will live and how often we will become sick mean a great deal to us. Yet, when we think of illness, we usually think of acute illness, the kind that responds to a treatment approach commonly known as the basic medical model. Broadly speaking, an acute illness usually has an abrupt onset, is limited in duration, and responds well to medical intervention such as technology, surgery, drugs, or other therapy.

Chronic illness is an entirely different phenomenon. A chronic illness or disability usually evolves more gradually. The condition may come and go episodically and have no definite duration or cure. Remission or death may not take place for a very long time. Pain and financial hardship accompany most chronic illnesses. Finally, the potentially devastating psychological and social impact of chronic conditions often demoralizes both the people with the condition and the family or friends who care for and interact with that person.

Some chronic medical problems are cancer, heart disease, arthritis, diabetes, lupus, fibromyalgia, chronic pain, emphysema, mental illness, and alcoholism and other drug addictions. Each violates one of the greatest human needs—the need to be in full control of all our physical, mental, and emotional functions and, thus, be able to act freely in seeking out life-fulfilling experiences. Hence, our response to chronic illness and its broader effects has important implications for the quality of our life.

Research has identified a number of common pathological responses to chronic conditions. Denial, self-absorption, depression, and anger are a few typical behavioral extremes.

These and other responses can drive normally caring people into a state of hostility and indifference. Self-defeating behavior associated with chronic conditions further injures the person who is ill and eventually takes its toll on everyone around.

Many people cope with chronic illness through "self-care," a term that includes everything from taking an active part in one's own primary medical care to attending self-help or mutual-help group activities. Nutrition, massage, acupuncture, and other complementary therapies are one avenue of self-care, which essentially means nearly everything people do for themselves to remain healthy or to treat illness.

Ultimately a person with a chronic illness benefits by becoming part of the solution, which can include getting together with other people who share the same problem. Groups exist for people affected by almost every kind of chronic physical or mental illness. Clearinghouses have been created to identify self-help groups in particular cities or regions throughout the country. These not-for-profit organizations not only help people with various needs to find an appropriate self-help group, but also assist them in starting new groups in their area. The following three self-help group clearinghouses can help:

The California Self-Help Center, Psychology Department, University of California, 405 Hilgard Ave., Los Angeles, CA 90024

The National Self-Help Clearinghouse, Graduate School and University Center of New York City, 33 West 42nd St., Room 620 N, New York, NY 10036

Self-Help Clearinghouse, Saint Clare's–Riverside Medical Center, Denville, NJ 07834

Another attribute of persons who live fully despite hardships is a willingness to work at doing so. Whatever the hurdles of the day—deteriorating health, ordinary problem solving, loss of intimacy with a spouse—these individuals pick up whatever they find in their path and act on it. They might encounter plenty of unpleasant feelings, but they work to assimilate those feelings and function as effective, whole persons.

One look at our addictive society testifies to the fact that we go to extraordinary lengths to avoid pain and eschew taking responsibility for ourselves. As a culture, we continue to try to find the easy way out, building elaborate fantasies in which to live or avoid meaningful contact with life. The psychiatrist and psychologist Carl Jung once said, "Neurosis is always a substitute for legitimate suffering." Our substitutes have sometimes become more painful than the legitimate suffering they were designed to avoid. Neither Eleanor nor Allie permitted any substitute for her legitimate movement toward reconciliation.

Owning her responsibilities played a critical role in Eleanor's progress toward wholeness. What she originally believed was the good life, a life of financial security, a solid marriage, and complete freedom from sickness and worry, has undergone a major reworking. Her husband, who suffered immensely under the stress of family upheaval, eventually left her, creating yet more pressure on Eleanor and her two small children. None of this set her so far off the path as to prevent her from attaining her goal of teaching others about chronic illness. Still, some days she bristles with a layer of anger that an able-bodied person doesn't have to accommodate. She has also had to make a decision, one she believes everyone with chronic illness has to make: What will she do about it? She can live with it and stretch every day to its maximum goodness, or she can mourn it and immerse herself in a sea of bitter resentment.

Eleanor chooses, for today, to make the best of it, though doing so doesn't eliminate bad days. It simply means she opts to say yes to life, and mean it. Having made that decision, she has taken over management of her own physical and spiritual nourishment. She began to write for others with chronic illness. She wrote to manufacturers and researched all the adaptive appliances and devices available to help her at home.

"What I'm trying to do is say to people, it is your right to have the best support you can find for yourself in order to live with your disease successfully. My illness," said Eleanor, "was *my* problem, and waiting around for someone else to solve it was going to be a long wait. Either I took a firm grip on my disease and my circumstances, or nothing would happen."

Allie exhibited many of the same qualities as Eleanor. She was often so physically restricted by lack of oxygen that even her simple daily routine became a mighty challenge. A modest job delivering newspapers to hospital patients provided her with some social stimulation and light exercise. Her godson helped her carry the largest paper bundles, but the rest she did alone, at her own measured pace. Chronic illness did slow Allie down, and it certainly drained her energy. But it didn't keep her from taking her parents to the dinner theater or from renting a pontoon boat with her family and going fishing.

Allie knew she could change at least some things by her own actions. She never said, "I can't . . ." "I couldn't . . . " "I have to . . . " "I had to . . . " Unlike many well individuals, she saw herself as one who had the power of choice. Despite her obvious limitations, she didn't permit her responses to be directed solely by external forces. She still shows up at music festivals, pushing other less able friends in wheelchairs. She gets out to Bible study meetings and collects Elvis Presley memorabilia. She opts to forge ahead, knowing that the farther she goes, the more endings and beginnings, the more births, the more pain, and the more joy she sees.

Even in the face of poor health, Eleanor and Allie find themselves excited about the future. They demonstrated a capacity to live with loss without being overwhelmed by loss. Hope is their ability to move out against resistance caused by anxiety over the unknown. Both women described joy as different from pleasure. Today they look back on their lives and understand that there was a time for everything.

CHAPTER 17

Looking for Meaning

❦

One in creation, you and I
kindred spirits
beloved
and bound together
untouched
by a world of limitations
walking together
upon the holy ground
of shared experience
knowing
we are human
and
this is enough

THE MESSAGE to come to labor and delivery arrived at about
four in the afternoon, an hour before the shift change. The social
worker had just interviewed the Morgan family and felt they might
benefit from a pastoral presence. Though the Morgans did not
belong to a local church, Mr. Morgan expressed curiosity about
meeting a woman minister.

"Mom is nearly full term, and her baby has died," reported
the social worker, highlighting some of the pertinent details in Mrs.
Morgan's chart. "She also has three small children at home and
probably suffers from serious psychiatric problems," she mumbled

offhandedly. Maybe bipolar disorder, schizophrenia, or borderline personality—or any of several other harrowing possibilities. The woman's reaction to her baby's death seemed "flat," according to others present at the nursing station. Most of the staff agreed that Mrs. Morgan had been joking oddly and that she failed to grasp the meaning of what was taking place in her life and her body.

A discussion then ensued about Mrs. Morgan's intellectual competence. The staff had given her some printed material about grief and loss, though they couldn't tell if she understood any of it, or even cared, for that matter. Perhaps the loss of this child was a relief to her, given the fact that she had a brood of very young children at home. The nurses and case managers continued to speculate about the situation. An unspoken question underlay their discussion: "Why would the Morgans continue to have children when Mrs. Morgan was so sick and she already had three youngsters under the age of four?"

I, too, wondered about the entire incident, as I observed the facial expressions around me. The expressions denoted everything from bewilderment to hostility and self-righteousness.

"How about the baby's father?" I asked. "Is he here?"

He was.

According to the staff, Mr. Morgan was behaving strangely, too. His strident voice and peculiar jokes made them uneasy. He dominated his wife, bossing her and hardly permitting her to answer questions for herself. Troubling, too, were his constant references to what he called his wife's medical mismanagement. He clearly thought that this might have contributed to their baby's death, and his questions were having a chilling effect on the various health professionals engaged in his wife's care.

Yet, though overbearing and odd, in some ways Mr. Morgan seemed quite supportive of his wife—quite sympathetic, and reassuring. A strong bond obviously existed between them. As I listened to the cacophony of opinions about the couple, it struck me that they were just that—individual opinions reflecting individual preferences, experiences, and comfort levels. The final diagnosis: Mr. Morgan talked too much, and he was . . . well, she was . . . that is, they were different. The social worker nodded in agreement.

I soon discovered that the Morgans were, indeed, different. They differed from me and from the rest of the staff in ways that hindered much meaningful contact. While the differences began at a racial level, they included profound social, cultural, educational, and financial contrasts. The Morgans embodied what could be described as a subculture of loss. White, middle-class, and educated, the rest of us exemplified a culture of privilege beyond the Morgans' experience or even comprehension.

The term "privilege" does not automatically jump off my tongue when I describe myself. Neutral or benign, perhaps, in the face of those who are culturally different but not privileged. To my knowledge, I've never intentionally wielded power over others. Nothing in my upbringing or education gave me any training in seeing myself as an oppressor. In fact, social justice ranks high on my list of priorities, a core value that has shaped my vocational call. But I also know that I spend most of my waking moments in the company of other whites, a relatively easy audience for me to identify and negotiate with. Rarely do I experience obstacles or setbacks that I can't transcend with a little determination and courage. In addition, I possess a convenient little bundle of provisions, tools that make my life uncommonly palatable—a passport, checkbook, credit cards, a home, a car that runs, health insurance, and, perhaps most significant, choices. This kind of privilege has little to do with my good intentions. A lifetime of good intentions did not make me any less privileged in the eyes of the people I was about to meet.

Mr. Morgan greeted me loudly with a predictable remark about never before having met a lady preacher. A thin veneer of jolly chatter barely concealed his anxiety and confusion. It wasn't long before he got to the point of his concern: "They say that our baby be dead for a long time," he announced, "maybe a month. Maybe it plans on risin' up like Lazarus! Do you think so, Reverend?"

He slapped his knee and, with a loud guffaw, beckoned to his wife, evidently granting her permission to chuckle with him over his icebreaking joke. She lay quietly in the bed, staring out the window, uncommitted to a discussion of any type. Mr. Morgan veered from one unrelated topic to another, regaling me with stories about everything from his tour of duty in the U.S. Army to the theology of Martin Luther.

I asked if they had friends I could call for them.

"No," he replied. "We keep pretty much to ourselves. I maybe leave the house to go to the grocery store, but I don't stay away long. We stick with each other and our kids most the time."

"How about family?" I pressed, hoping to identify someone who might lend support. Mr. Morgan's parents had died some time ago. Mrs. Morgan's mother lived in Arkansas, but didn't have a telephone—or much else, for that matter. Neither of them knew how to reach any other relatives.

"No, we don't need to call no family," said Mr. Morgan. "We can take care of this ourselves."

Soon I learned that the Morgans had left Arkansas six months ago. They were heading for Canada when their dilapidated car broke down on the freeway. A highway patrolman arrived and, upon discovering that they had no automobile insurance, collected a $300 fine from them. The encounter left the family broke and marooned in the Twin Cities. When we met, they had already moved several times in search of a safe neighborhood for their children.

"A baby always loves you, you know. Like, I know that a baby needs me to take care of it. I like that, don't you? I'm scared," she said.

"A lady preacher. Well now, ain't that something? It would be good if you stayed with my wife while she has that baby. You know, my sister lost a baby once. And my wife's mama lost twins. Hell, we've lost a lot of children, now that I think about it. Yes, you could be a comfort to her when she has that baby."

Loss of power. Loss of identity. Loss of life.

"Is there anyone you would like to see, or anything I could do for you? I've never had a child die. I don't know what it's like to be who you are or where you are. I'm sorry."

"That baby ain't never done nothin' wrong, has it? God is gonna welcome that baby, isn't He? 'Course He will. I know it couldn't be no other way. I mean, what's that baby ever done wrong anyhow? 'Course God is gonna do that."

Loss of dignity. Loss of hope. Loss of dreams.

"You know, the other day I come out to get in the car and the horn started to honk. Just like that. It was the day my wife found out that the baby died. That darn horn be honking all the way downtown. People kep' lookin at me, and I kep' holdin' my hands up in the air—like this—so they could see I wasn't doin' it myself. It was doin' it itself. Craziest thing I ever did see. I think maybe that baby's spirit was right in that car, don't you know? That be it. I know it. That baby's spirit was in that car telling us it was gonna be just fine up there in heaven. Do you think so, Reverend?"

Loss of access. Loss of privacy. Loss of connection.

"Mr. Morgan, I was wondering if the three of us could hold hands for a few minutes."

He struggled out of his chair and made his way to the bedside where he took his wife's hand and then mine. We stood motionless against a backdrop of fetal monitors and rush-hour traffic. Gripped by my own inadequacy, I offered a halting prayer of encouragement . . . for all of us. Tears slowly slipped down Mr. Morgan's cheeks. Mrs. Morgan kept her silent vigil, seemingly trying to summon the courage to give birth to her dead child.

We tightened our grips on one another's hands, a spontaneous gesture that found me at once understanding everything and nothing.

It was but a mere hesitation, a suspended moment in space, when we three said yes to a life briefly shared and broken. Wordlessly we acknowledged the fragile and precious thread that knitted us together, suspended in time and creation, a merging of kindred spirits never to be separated by a world of human limitations.

WHEN SOMEONE DIES

The prospect of being with another person who has recently lost someone to death can be both difficult and frightening. None of us comes fully prepared to face another's grief; in fact, most of us come ill prepared and tend to stumble despite our best intentions. There are no easy recipes or formulas, and each situation is unique. However, with a little thought and care, anyone can contribute in a positive way to a difficult situation. First—and, perhaps, most important—show up. Once you choose to be with that person, begin by simply listening and letting pain be pain without trying to fix it.

When someone has been bereaved, or has received a life-threatening diagnosis, our presence can produce a number of healing effects. We can help to move another toward healing when we:

> Embody a message that the individual or family does not
> have to go through this crisis alone
> Facilitate their acceptance of the full range of their emo-
> tional responses
> Support their development of meaningful connections with
> others
> Enable them to begin grieving in healthy ways
> Offer them assurance that life does go on and that you will
> accompany them in this process

A key figure in the world of hospitals is the stranger. Whether we're learning about a patient's belief system or launching a physician's treatment plan, a hospital always finds us in new lands, working among strangers. Often we become intimate strangers, venturing into the unknown together, away from the realms of safety, comfort, and security. A hospital setting can test

The Words We Use Truly Matter

Friends, relatives, and even health care professionals tend to feel helpless and inadequate when encountering those who have experienced a loss. It is important for everyone to remember that words of support and encouragement can contribute in a very helpful way to the healing process. For example:

Ask the person to tell her or his story and describe the events surrounding this loss.

Acknowledge that you don't know exactly what the person feels like.

Ask if he wants you to call someone to be with him; encourage him to ask for help, and perhaps, help him to make a list of what he needs from friends.

Ask if she needs more information to help her understand the situation or make decisions.

Use honest and respectful words near to her experience, not abstract terms and euphemisms; help to validate the person's feelings.

Don't be afraid of awkward silence; your presence offers comfort, even without words.

one's faith and convictions on many levels. And sometimes such a setting brings us new faith, especially when a stranger steps into our lives and shines a new light to help us see.

Parker J. Palmer, a writer and a professor of sociology at Georgetown University, describes the stranger as a bearer of truth that might not otherwise have been received. "We often need the stranger's line of vision to help us see straight," he explains. "For example, each of us has potentials and limitations which become invisible to us and those near us; we cannot see the forest for the trees. But when the stranger comes along and looks at us afresh, without bias or preconception, those qualities may quickly become apparent."[1] A startling truth that came to light the day I met the Morgan family.

CHAPTER 18

An Issue of Faith

❧❦

We light a candle in gratitude
for the gift of children.
May its light surround this home and those who dwell here.
May your healing presence be theirs,
this night,
tomorrow,
and always.
Amen

THE YOUNG PARENTS *placed their dying son amidst a pile of*
pillows and stuffed toys in the middle of the living room floor.
On this sultry late-summer evening, their tiny home overflowed
with people and signs of love. The kitchen table overflowed with
casseroles and cookies, while pets and small children galloped
around the backyard. Three-year-old Carter had been diagnosed
nearly two years earlier with a particularly deadly brain tumor.
His treatment encompassed the most aggressive cancer protocols
available. Though statistics showed that most children with this
kind of tumor lived barely as long as the treatment lasted, Carter
had defied those odds. Not only did he continue to live in relatively
good health, he enjoyed a life of immeasurable quality and sub-
stance. However, this night, with medical options having run their
course, everyone suspected that love and faith provided the only
"medicines" that sustained Carter.

Brothers, sisters, aunts, and uncles had joyfully participated in the little boy's treatment and care. Neighbors and teachers joined in as well. Birthday parties, school visits, trips to the zoo, baseball games, and a pilgrimage to a holy place in France made up a series of simple and elaborate events that moved life along. No matter where he traveled, Carter charmed everyone he met. Prayer chains extended across the country and over the Internet. Healing services, special masses, and potluck fund-raisers—these and other collective efforts by concerned friends and strangers upheld Carter and his family for nearly two years. Now, with time running out, this large Irish Catholic family gathered their brood to renew their commitments to their God and one another.

Having abandoned the search for a satisfactory or rational explanation of their child's disease, Carter's parents now concentrated on living creatively in the presence of this aggressive tumor. In keeping with this decision, they decided to plan a home liturgy honoring their wise and irresistible son. In preparation for the service, I asked each member of the extended family, including the smallest children, to bring a gift. It was not to be a purchased gift, but something such as photos, poems, or handmade scrapbooks to share with Carter. I also asked that each gift be accompanied by an individual promise that they would like to make to Carter.

Though countless prayers had not eliminated Carter's tumor, this family had managed to transform the quality of their inner or spiritual world as they accompanied their youngest child in his walk toward death. For them, faith became a real revolution of consciousness, an inner transformation that enabled them to see their circumstances and their son from a new perspective. Faith became, in their eyes and hearts, a life viewed from the standpoint of love.

Carter's mother often talked about faith. She spoke not as someone blind to reality but as a woman who trusted the importance of all human life, short or long. From teachers and homemakers to grandparents to a little boy with a bad tumor, everyone mattered to her. For her, not only do our lives make a difference but also we

*can actually change the world. After all, she had watched Carter
change the world—their world and that of everyone else he met.
Forced to look hard at her own priorities, she concluded that none
of us creates change by struggling to get to the top of the heap or
fighting over who should lead and who should follow. Our lives
make a difference not because we have negotiated our way to the
head of the success train. We aren't called, after all, to be successful but to be faithful—to care for one another, to seek justice and
peace, and to recognize the value and dignity of each person.*

Without this point of view, we tend to look for security in the
number and quality of the objects that surround us. We begin to
value only those things that make us relevant. We are what we
do—important when we do important things, intelligent when
we say something intelligent. We are valuable only if we do
something perceived as valuable. In this kind of world, it is
extremely difficult to have faith that a vital, divine energy flows
through the veins of ordinary family routines, especially when
these routines involve caring for a dying child. According to
Carter's mother, their family had been blessed, not by good luck
but in their capacity to live in the moment with Carter.

Faith, for this family, required that they appreciate every
passing hour with its tentative promises and fleeting light. They
saw an earthly realism in the conviction that we ought to make
the most of the moment—to live one day at a time, as the
popular phrase goes. The ability to live creatively in the present helped them remain emotionally whole through Carter's
final days.

So what, actually, is faith? One might call it the thrust of the
soul into a future always hidden. Faith also means the anticipation of future good and the ability to accept life with gratitude,
even a life darkened with uncertainty and pain. Faith, for Carter's family, consisted of a belief system that could adapt to all
that life dished out.

WHY A PATIENT'S SPIRITUAL AND CULTURAL BELIEF SYSTEM MATTERS

Loss is truly a spiritual issue. Though loss is an obvious by-product of illness, some losses are less visible than others. Families and patients report a wide range of losses: independence; power; privacy; dignity; daily routines; money; control; identity; dreams; marriages and other relationships; jobs; function; and security. In my experience, families with strong religious and cultural belief systems tend to draw strength from those beliefs when faced with a significant loss. It seems that spirituality and cultural belief systems

Help people cope with illness

Provide a source of hope in the face of death or illness

Furnish practical resources to help patients and families contend with sickness—for example, prayer, social support, and rituals help create order and structure for both patients and their caregivers

For patients and families, it is always important to find some meaning in the experience of illness. This family's faith allowed them to place Carter in the hands of a larger authority, a source of creation that released them to a new form of living and integration. It allowed them to continue thriving in the face of uncertainty.

But we live in a world that doesn't like this kind of uncertainty. Since the Enlightenment, we have demanded answers. We want to repair things and find certain remedies. We try to place things in orderly compartments and strive for black-and-white precision and clarity. We long for proof. The age in which we live is full of attempted proofs of all kinds, including proof of the divine. Erich von Daniken claims that God is really a fleet of

Contribute to patient and family compliance with medical
care
Give physicians helpful history and diagnostic information
while enriching the quality of their medical practice

It is not necessary for a doctor to share a patient's spiritual or
cultural beliefs. It is only necessary to

Know that these beliefs are of value
Understand and respect the patient's or family's belief
systems, since such systems tend to remain securely
in place and resist change
Know that you don't have to believe in miracles to appre-
ciate the strength of the human spirit
Reflect honestly on your own fears and resistance
Realize that you cannot fix everything but you always have
something of value to offer your patients
Be prepared to listen and admit that you have no answers
Accept that you are human and that this is enough

intergalactic visitors. Huge industries suggest that God is really
perfect health or fitness. Pathologists from the Mayo Clinic tried
to prove that Jesus died from hanging, and modern science continues to examine the Shroud of Turin to find out if it was really
the shroud Jesus' body was wrapped in for burial. In an age that
demands proof, Carter's family chose the route of good medical
treatment combined with a simple lived faith.

So, on a sticky summer evening in a modest, working-class
home, we all knew how many lives Carter had touched. He, too,
demonstrated a remarkably clear faith. His time with us was
very important, and one of the reasons it was important was that
he made us listen. He made us pay attention. We felt privileged
to learn from him about courage, and about joy and fun. While

we fussed with our daily deadlines and self-inflicted schedules, Carter showed us how sacred the daily plans of a little boy could be: going to the park, throwing a ball, lying in bed with his brothers jouncing in and out, on top of him, on top of one another. While we anxiously tried to gain control over our tomorrows and next weeks, Carter gave new meaning to living in the moment. His abbreviated life provided an example of acceptance and gratitude for what is—not bitterness about what is missing or unfair or wrong.

Finally, toward the end of his life, at a time when well-intentioned people sometimes slip away from the dying, the opposite occurred. People pressed even closer to Carter, lest they miss some treasured lesson. Their instincts were correct. We all felt both honored to know him and destined to learn from him.

According to a certain philosopher, those who do not have faith are forced to be happy about the little things of life, but sad about the ultimate realities. On the other hand, those who believe are more willing to accept pain along with the joy of daily living, because their vision is permeated with hope. I would add to this that believers are those who can live fully in the face of darkness and not always insist on hard-and-fast answers. There is a receptivity and malleability inherent in faith that allow one to maintain an openness to possibilities. These very qualities Carter and his family left with each of us who knew them.

CHAPTER 19

Hospitality as Gift

❦❦

THE TIME ALWAYS COMES when someone asks, "Why?" Nurses, physicians, social workers, and all those who encounter others' pain eventually must face the question, "Why is there needless suffering in the world? Why do innocent children die? Where is the so-called God of love and compassion in the midst of our cynicism and discouragement? For what can we hope? How do we replenish the dry and brittle souls of others when we feel so depleted?"

For all the colleagues and friends who have asked me, "Where is God's light hiding in my time of need?" I offer the following story.

Long ago, one deep, dark night, a small party of powerful gods met to discuss a frightening revelation—a threat of such scale that it endangered their very survival as gods. It seemed that, while they had been reclining upon their ample backsides, boasting of their admirable achievements, a rumor began circulating among the mortals. The rumor claimed that they, mere mortals, also held the potential for divinity. Deeply disturbed at this career-threatening breakthrough, the gods made haste to convene a blue-ribbon task force to study the matter.

The impressive guest list said it all. Fertility gods, war gods, sports gods, celebrity gods—the works—every majestic mover and

115

supreme shaker whose reputation stood to suffer from this looming disaster received a summons.

The meeting day arrived, and delegates of every celestial order appeared. First came registration and refreshments . . . a bit of small talk. Quickly, however, the standard schmoozing gave way to a clamorous cacophony framed by one burning question:

"What are we going to do about these ungrateful boors who call themselves mortals?"

"Who do they think they are?" snorted an irritable investment god. "For years I've heard nothing but whine, whine, whine. 'Buy this.' 'Sell that.' 'Maybe mutual funds.' 'No, make it wheat futures.' I can't remember when they haven't been making some kind of demand. Now it looks as if they want to compete with us, for heaven's sake. They might be tiresome to work with, but if mortals ever do find this divine spark, I could be out of business. We all could be standing in the royal unemployment lines!"

"You're absolutely right!" roared a defense god. "A discovery like this could spell supremely slashed budgets and heavenly hiring freezes. Why, imagine what would happen if they figured out how to get along without us . . . or with each other, god forbid! You know the old chestnut 'No bombs, no budgets.' That means downsized operations. Maybe even early retirements. If this spark gets out of the bag, we can say good-bye golf games and hello quality improvement consultants.

"No doubt about it, we need to settle down and figure out where on earth we can hide the spark of divinity so that mortals never get their hands on it."

Ideas whirled about the conference hall—wild and complicated schemes. Gods whose social paths rarely crossed now huddled together, oddly linked through a common fear for their future security. What a throng of stewing sovereigns they made.

Unfortunately, their rank outshone their cleverness, for none came up with a solution that the others could agree upon.

"Upstarts," grumbled a football deity. "They have no idea just how tricky this god business can be when it lands in the wrong hands."

Everyone nodded, appreciative of his discerning insight.

The day passed with no sign of a solution. Twilight seeped across the frozen landscape. Currents of life retired to their silent roots, waiting for winter and some solution to the immediate crisis. The gods mused. Beleaguered delegates reconvened, pinch-faced and pale, to tick off a lackluster list of ideas.

"How about hiding this spark of divinity in an oyster at the bottom of the sea?" offered one. "Or perhaps in a distant galaxy?"

"No, no, no," growled an IRS god. "Why, in no time, some diver or astronaut will discover it and steal it away."

"How about inside a smoldering volcano?" proposed another.

"Or in an eagle's nest high upon a mountain peak?" advised a third. "Perhaps among the bunchberries that cover the forest floor?"

Disapproving murmurs followed each suggestion. At last they gave up and prepared to leave. Suddenly an elderly woman, a Hearthkeeper, raised her hand tentatively to report that she might have the answer to the question of where to hide the divine spark.

"What is it?" demanded the chief executive god, who, by this time, had a migraine and wanted to go home. "Speak up, madam."

The Hearthkeeper rose to her feet with a certain grace and rather floated to the front of the conference hall. Far less flamboyant than the other delegates, she wore a simple woolen tunic, with a linen shawl about her shoulders. With her silver hair secured in an amber clasp, she exuded both mystery and wisdom. She was known throughout the countryside not for theatrical, godlike acts but for her capacity to listen. Most of the other gods found her slightly strange, as she always seemed preoccupied with the well-being of humans. Though none of the gods had ever actually caught her speaking to a mortal, some suspected her of giving away trade secrets.

The woman whispered her proposal to the chief executive god. He brightened. Normally he might have dismissed a Hearthkeeper's idea, but he had nothing better to offer—and besides, he could hardly keep from admiring her cleverness.

He shared her idea with his assistant, who actually laughed out loud with delight. The gloom lifted slightly from the room as, one by one, the guests passed the Hearthkeeper's suggestion among themselves. Nonetheless, even in their excitement, they spoke in a whisper for fear that some gate-crashing mortal might overhear.

"It's perfect," crowed the defense god jubilantly. "Why, even heat-seeking missiles couldn't find it there. No one will find the spark of divinity now. We need never again contend with those brazen humans overstepping their authority."

With that, the delegates voted unanimously in favor of the Hearthkeeper's idea and then departed from the convention.

A year later, in the month of December, two men plodded along a dark and lonely road in the northern territory. They walked without words, staring sadly at the night sky. Snow drifted about their feet in soft meringue peaks. Disillusioned and brokenhearted, they leaned into the wind. The winter landscape lay unadorned except by a frozen sky. They heard no music beyond the bitter wind. The night bore them only icy tears. They had been searching for a divine spark, but tonight they abandoned hope. Now the men simply longed for home and a warm fire.

An elderly woman stood alone at the roadside. Bundled in a simple woolen tunic, she watched from beneath her shawl. The travelers moved slowly, driving themselves onward with thoughts of a warm hearth. When they came within hearing distance, she called to them pleasantly:

"Who are you, and what brings you out on such a night as this?"

"We're weary mortals," called back the younger man through the darkness. "We've been searching. We have combed the valleys

and hillsides, convinced that we would find a divine spark, a light
of implication."

"But why do you seek such a light?" queried the woman.

"Because we have become impoverished by our affluence and
broken by our own powerlessness," lamented the older man. "We
hunger for hope and yearn for reconciliation. We are overburdened
by tension and confused by the world's empty promises. We need
such a light to show us the way."

The woman inquired further, "What makes you think this
divine spark exists? And tell me, too, what would you do with it
should you find it?"

The older man continued his bitter repining, as if he hadn't
heard her. "Snow falls now on our path. We have watched the skies
for signs. We have wandered the roads of our past, questioning
what we might have done differently to lead us to this wondrous
spark. We have traveled through streets of violence and oppression
in hope of kindling a new flame in our hearts. We envisioned healing and peace."

The woman reached out to receive their sorrow and pressed it
to her heart. Then she asked if they would accompany her to her
hearth. The exhausted and freezing men agreed, and the three set
off together into the night of discovery.

"Do you know that night is the birth of all things?" the woman
asked her two companions. "Night wears a mantle of snow; shiver-
ing in the darkness, it watches and waits. Winter is a waiting season and a time of breakthroughs."

The men listened but did not understand. They walked in
silence until they came to the woman's hut. She invited them in
to warm by her fire and refresh themselves.

"Break bread with me," she implored. "Let your strength
return before you continue your search."

Inside the hut, encircled by warmth, the travelers accepted a
bit of cheese and hot tea from the woman while they dried their
clothes near her hearth. Her simple cottage boosted their spirits,
a cozy respite from their heavy burdens and paralyzing cold.

Meanwhile, the woman busied herself preparing a parcel of food, which she wrapped in her linen shawl. She helped the men into their coats and wished them well as they set out for home.

"This should see you through the night," she said, handing them the small bundle. "Blessings on you and yours," she called warmly behind them as they disappeared into the dark.

Near dawn, the men came to a small village. Exhausted from fighting the wind and snow, they took shelter in a barn. They settled themselves into a mound of straw and thought about the strange woman. They thought also about their failed search for the spark of divinity.

"We have not accomplished anything that we set out to do." The older man sighed. "All the good intentions. All the dreams and plans. All our hopes for success have failed. It just doesn't seem fair."

In thoughtful stillness, they contemplated the events of the past months. At last, the young man pulled the woman's bundle from beneath his coat to see what she had given them to eat. He laid the contents upon the straw to share with his friend: a piece of cheese, a loaf of bread, some dried apples, and a few hazelnuts. Beneath the food lay an envelope secured by an amber clasp, the kind a woman would wear to secure her long hair.

They ate, while the older man removed the amber clasp and opened the envelope. He examined the contents carefully. On a single piece of parchment was written the following:

Break this bread and think of me
A sage who has lived enough to see
That peace and fairness and love are real
For those who hear and forgive and feel
Who keep the hearth and tend the meal
Who warm a space for others to heal
Who nurture a child and care for the sick
And seek to be just in all that they pick
Who lighten the dark that others might see

And think with their heart and learn just to be
Who know how to laugh and know how to grieve
And celebrate life, both its pain and reprieve.

To you who have searched every place far and near
You now need to know that there's nothing to fear
For all that is well will be well from now on
With you who have wandered and struggled anon.
For lo, as you looked everywhere for the spark
The light that you seek lives right in your heart.

HEAVENLY WHOLE WHEAT BREAD

Perhaps nothing enhances the quality of our lives more than preparing and eating good food. And nothing offers a richer example of shared life than bread. Whether we speak of bread in terms of food, money, community, or comfort, it enjoys an expansive history of association with nurturing and healing.

2 cups lukewarm milk
2 packets active dry yeast
⅓ cup honey
3 cups whole wheat flour
1 egg, beaten
2 teaspoons salt
½ teaspoon nutmeg
½ cup butter
3–4 cups unbleached all-purpose flour

POUR milk into mixing bowl. Stir in 1 teaspoon honey; add yeast and whole wheat flour and cover loosely. Leave for 20 minutes. Mix in the rest of the honey, the egg, salt, nutmeg, butter, and 3 to 3½ cups of the all-purpose flour. Mix until dough begins to pull away from sides of the bowl. Place the dough on a board and knead for 8 to 10 minutes, until smooth and elastic. Divide

into two, shape loaves, and place in two greased bread pans.
Let rise until doubled in bulk, about 1 to 1 1/2 hours.

BAKE in preheated 350-degree oven for 35 to 40 minutes. Share
one loaf with a friend.

ADVOCATE   *Advocating means supporting or acting as an ally,
a champion, a helper, a defender, a benefactor and sustainer.
All patients deserve advocates to help them through their health
crisis. All who are frail, vulnerable, poor, or alone need advocates to help them mobilize the resources they require to protect
or restore their health. To advocate for another is to offer the
prospect of renewed life and vitality.*

CHAPTER 20

Where Cure and Healing Meet

❧❧

THE TERMS "cure" and "healing" signify two distinct avenues to the same end: becoming whole. Used in this context, "cure" pertains to specific acts of scientific intervention. "Healing," on the other hand, points to a set of possibilities that all of us, not just health care professionals, can bring to a seemingly incurable situation. While a healing approach might not always change a medical outcome or prevent a loss, it can improve our own or another's sense of well-being. A healing presence encompasses gifts that each of us already possesses, gifts that can brighten even the darkest hour.

This human capacity for healing came sharply into focus one morning during a presentation I made to a grief support group for older adults. I somehow thought the subject, loss as a spiritual dilemma, would capture the attention of everyone present; however, the room seemed almost overwhelmingly silent rather than open to discussion. Everyone simply stared back at me, their fixed expressions edged in melancholy. The silence set the tone for the opening activity, led by a therapist.

Her therapeutic game required that each member of the group pick a flower that characterized what he or she felt like at this hour on this particular morning. Once everyone had selected a flower, the therapist invited them to describe its characteristics and explain how these characteristics related to their own current life experience.

The group members made fascinating though sometimes heart-breaking choices. One woman chose a rose, reporting that sharp thorns that discouraged people from coming near her had over-whelmed her beauty. Friends and family either avoided her or wore gloves to protect themselves from the painful experience of touching her.

A man in his late sixties described himself as ivy, once robust and lush, and now cut back to a smaller self. He felt he had been subjected to relentless pruning until, today, only a woody and lifeless stump remained. This man had recently left his job of thirty years.

The therapist proceeded around the room until arriving at the last member, an attractive though expressionless woman of about sixty-five. Straight-backed and silent, she had not said a thing since the session began. I felt certain she would say nothing now.

Her first words caused a few people to grimace with embar-rassment. Papers rustled and backsides shifted uncomfortably. The woman struggled to tell a peculiar story that nobody under-stood. The therapist encouraged her to continue while others fidgeted.

"The dark," she repeated emphatically, "the one that grew in the dark."

Eventually, with the help of the therapist and several other group members, the woman was able to articulate a previous presentation and identify the flower she felt like. A narcissus . . . the flower that begins life in utter darkness. The following tale reflects the woman's discovery and the first steps of her return journey "home."

The Narcissus

A child once visited a garden with her grandmother.

The two of them wandered hand in hand among the ancient beech trees, narrow paths banked with foxglove, antique roses, and delicate Turk's-cap lilies. The old woman told her granddaughter of many mysterious and healing properties of flowers. She spoke of roots and petals crushed into secret potions, exotic balms, magic elixirs, and bewitching perfumes.

Eventually they came upon a willow basket filled with flower bulbs. The grandmother invited the girl to select one of the bulbs so that she might take it home and plant it in her own garden. After inspecting the snarled clump of roots, the girl made her choice and slipped it into the pocket of her dress.

"That is a very special bulb you've chosen," said her grandmother. "It's called a narcissus, and you must cultivate it with great care in order to extract all of its beauty and healing power. The first thing you must do when you get home is hide it in a dark place, and leave it there until it begins to sprout. Only when the bulb has sent out roots can you plant it among the rest of the flowers."

The child thought this rather odd, but promised her grandmother she would do as she instructed.

After placing the bulb in a mixture of moss and damp clay, they set it out of sight on a cellar shelf. However, the little girl could not resist opening the door every once in a while to see if the narcissus had started to grow. Every once in a while soon became every hour and sometimes even more. Each morning she sprang from her bed, raced down the steps to the dark root cellar, and peered through the shadows, hoping to see some sign of life. Each day brought greater disappointment than the last.

She sulked. She cried. She wailed to her grandmother, convinced that she had brought home a dead bulb. The old woman listened politely but only counseled patience. One morning, while the household still slept, the child crept down to the cellar and removed the bulb from its hiding place. She washed the clay

SEARCHING FOR MEANING IN THE MIDST OF CHAOS

A crisis in health often sets in motion events and feelings that often include losses, dread, and a sense of helplessness. At the center of this chaos, individuals and families struggle to make sense of the illness by seeking to, once again, find meaning and hope in their lives.

The following inventory can help to reveal that elusive spiritual meaning in the midst of a health crisis. The questions encompass the challenges, opportunities, and spiritual qualities that enable people to rise above human suffering and reestablish peace and order in their lives. By attending to these questions, caregivers, those living with a chronic illness, and anyone who has experienced major losses can potentially reshape their experience of illness and their capacity to hope.

> Name some of the dreams you had in your twenties/
>   forties/sixties.
> Have you realized some of these dreams? Which ones?
> How do you feel about your inability to fulfill all of these
>   dreams?
> What do you presently dream of and hope for?
> What makes it difficult for you to let go and move on?

from its smooth onionlike skin and examined the surface with a reading glass. Nothing.

Finally, after weeks of watching and wishing, the child gave up hope. Surely she would never see her narcissus bloom. Bored with waiting and certain that the bulb would never grow, she stopped checking on it. How silly, she thought, to think that such an ugly little thing could ever turn into something beautiful, especially in the dark.

If you had only one year left to live, how would you spend
    your time?
Do you have important relationships in your life that need
    healing?
What aspects of those relationships make it difficult for
    you to forgive yourself or the other person?
When was the last time you forgave yourself or another?
When was the last time you felt comfortable and at home
    with yourself?
What do you yearn for?
What do you hope for?
List ten things that nurture your spirit.
When was the last time you engaged in these activities?
What is your image of God, or of the Holy?
How has your perception of life changed as a result of your
    illness, loss, or physical diminishment?
Do you feel you have an adequate support system? Do you
    have a space in which you can be vulnerable and
    unjudged?
Do you feel you have adequate spiritual support?
What is the most important thing you have learned in life?
If you are a caregiver, what do you think others expect of
    you? What do you expect of yourself?
Do you want to be well?

*Then, one day, her grandmother called to her from the
bottom of the cellar steps. "Look here," said the old woman
brightly. "Something seems to have happened to your bulb."*

*Her granddaughter gasped in disbelief when she saw the
little pot of soil. Something, indeed, had happened. The bulb
had sprouted. From its top protruded a soft green nub and
underneath, a thick clump of roots. Sure enough, the narcissus
was alive.*

It grew quickly then, flourishing in the dark just as her grandmother had promised. Soon the child moved it from the cellar to a spot in the garden bed reserved for the first flowers of spring.

To this day, the little bulb continues to thrive, though each winter it retires to a dark and mysterious place from which it draws healing energy so that it might bloom the following spring.

As in our human lives, real growth often takes place in darkness. Darkness is where simple wishes are transformed into enduring faith. God and healing meet in the unlit corners of the human heart. It is the winter days and long nights of our lives that invite us to send down roots, to grow in courage and hope. When we accept this invitation to wait patiently in our darkness, we accept the possibility of a new quest toward a season of hope.

CHAPTER 21

Maturity Points Us toward Acceptance

❧❦

For everything there is a season and a time for every matter under heaven.

—Ecclesiastes 3:1

IN THE HEBREW BIBLE, the book of Ecclesiastes is called Qoheleth. The purpose of this wisdom figure, Qoheleth, was not so much to teach about God, but rather to tell what he had discovered about life and what humans might gain from life. He set out his viewpoints on the value of life and outlined a doctrine of opposites, like two currents flowing in the same stream. Woven into the fabric of Qoheleth's reflections are much larger, more persistent questions: What is life worth? What real value does life have to offer? How do we come to grips with the mystery and the ambiguity of life? And what about sickness and suffering and all those shadowy conditions that we can't fix but can only experience?

Qoheleth asked what one might call the big "religious" questions, the ones that have endured throughout human history and that, at some point or another, most of us ask.

Such queries arose one early spring morning at the breakfast table in a small western Wisconsin town. A woman named Irene described what it was like to watch her father grow old.

They sat at opposite ends of the kitchen table, father and daughter, comfortable with the long silences that yawned and stretched between them in the early morning. The previous week's unseasonably warm weather had been good for his health. Traditionally, these first weeks of April found them watching together for sure signs of the earth reaching toward life. A soft transition from winter to a season of more kindly disposition helped him regain some of the stamina necessary to make it through another year. For the next few months, they would be free of bone-chilling squalls of snow and sleet. No more plummeting thermometers, as winter had finally relaxed its brittle grip and given way to a changing quality of light. A pale thin sun bathed the early morning sky in anticipation of change.

Migrating redpolls converged on a chunk of thawing suet that hung from a linden tree. Winter-shabby gray squirrels scuttled among the autumn's leftover maple leaves. A few fiddleheads poked cautiously through the moist ground cover at the edges of the woods. The human heart has always responded to the certainty of spring. A birthing process had begun. Though it would take weeks for the growing season to officially arrive, the signs were already fixed in place.

He wore his flannel pajama bottoms and an undershirt. A shower of blood vessels fell across the paper-thin skin of his forearms. Years of using steroids to keep his emphysema at bay had taken a heavy toll, both on his moods and on his physical appearance. Nonetheless, this would be a good day.

She watched him methodically ingest an array of capsules and prepare to use the inhaler that would relieve his labored breathing. He paused briefly between each dose of pills to observe, with obvious comfort, his dog in the backyard poking among piles of old leaves and branches. The dog also seemed to recognize familiar *clues that announced an arrival of a new season. Raising her head to the breeze, she basked in the earthen smells and sounds that rekindle life in the upper Midwest.*

All living creatures respond to the earth's seasonal transformations. Hibernating and migrating patterns, social and working patterns—all of these demonstrate the influence of our earth recreating itself. Research into northern winters even suggests that people become more depressed during months when there are few hours of daylight. The seasons influence the way we work and live, what we wear, the foods we eat, and the homes we build. We respond in countless ways to the cycle of the seasons and the qualities of the earth.

Our interest in the earth is no accident or fleeting trend. We have a vital need to be close to the earth and to all her expressions. It is critical that we learn to protect and preserve her precious resources and fragile beauty. She is vulnerable as we are vulnerable. Even our vast resources of technology and science do not make us less vulnerable or less apt to get old and sick. We are born from the earth and nurtured by her, and we will ultimately return to her. We live on an island home in a vast expanse of interstellar space, galaxies, suns, and planets. We are assailable. To say that human life unfolds much as the earth and her seasons unfold isn't enough.

According to Irene, the man sitting across the table from her embodied vast wisdom and courage, gained through years of living. For the better part of a century he had enjoyed a fine adventure as well as a brilliant law career. Both were punctuated by a host of personal and intellectual accomplishments and a hearty ability to laugh, especially at himself.

No way could his life be reduced to a simple exercise of growing up and ripening. Maturity such as this represented more than physical readiness for harvest. It included an inner growth toward

wholeness. It brought to light a strength that was able to tran-
scend the past, live in the present, and engage fully and deeply in
a world that includes suffering, sickness, and old age with all its
diminishments.

Contrary to what we might have learned, human maturity doesn't just happen. It anticipates the presence of certain assets such as a community of friends, family, colleagues, and others who function as nurturers and sensors of one another's values. A mature person like this man has learned to consider his life experience through the eyes of his spiritual self, a quality that helps him not only to survive but also to interpret the events that surround him as part of a larger, more meaningful whole. This clarity of vision influences everything from the way he celebrates to the ways he finds support in his pain and illness.

Listening to Irene's commentary on her father helped me understand what kind of grit it must have taken for him to move from vital, productive years, through a difficult transition into retirement, and at last into the final leg of his journey into old age.

This particular morning marked the way of his last passage into
a quieter and delicate time. No longer did he engage in courtroom
gymnastics or wade the Brule River with his fly rod and creel.
Gone were the days when he scoured Bayfield County with his
favorite hunting dog flushing pheasant. He couldn't see so well
anymore. He couldn't hear too well, either. Some days he felt just
plain lousy and let everyone know it. Some days he slept too much
and groused about everything.

On other days he pulled on his long underwear, rounded up the
dog, and drove to Chetek to buy homemade sausage from a farmer
he had known for years. On another afternoon he put in his hear-
ing aid and spent a few hours conversing with his grandchildren.
Or he rustled up a few remaining cohorts and set out for a lunch

*spot where they regaled one another with exaggerated stories about
Prohibition, deer hunting, and basement poker games.*

*In Irene's eyes, if ever there was a life worth living, it surely
was her father's. On all fronts, professionally and personally, he
challenged life, made friends with life, poked fun at life, and
finally, with fearless dignity, accepted aspects of life and health
over which he had no control. Even then, as he stood face-to-face
with the end of his life, he continued to savor its richness.*

*This was not a man who sought publicity or fame. He never
needed to travel far or accumulate a larger worldly experience.
In fact, he preferred to stay home. Surely he appreciated the success of his achievements, yet his real success lay in his ability to
learn and to change when change was necessary. His significant
accomplishments came in making substantial legal decisions and
in his splendid sense of humor.*

*Never did he stop learning, she explained, and never did he
give up a chance to move closer to becoming the person he was
meant to be, even if that person had nothing better to do that day
than ride his exercise bicycle on an imaginary trip to Bloomer.*

Aging and illness invite us to move inward in search of the
things that won't fall to the ground or decay like last fall's leaves.
They pull us toward an interior, spiritual light that will not fade.
This inward journey of the human spirit is not just a goal or
level of achievement that we work to attain. It is a process, ever
moving, ever changing.

Like the venerable old man's, our spiritual life arises from
our human life. It reflects the way we live and interpret the mystery that surrounds us. It includes the ways we maintain traditions, how we recover from loss, and how we find reconciliation
with events and others. Spirituality encompasses our political
and social behavior as well as the gifts we share with others. It
encompasses the outlook we have on our work and the attitude
we assume about our time on earth. It cries out with a message

of liberation and includes specific acts of freeing ourselves from .
restrictions of space, time, and matter.

Movement toward acceptance of life evolves from years of
searching, learning, and unlearning. It takes decades of self-
discovery and new beginnings. Like Irene's father, we learn great
truths only in the course of time, and usually by looking backward at them. We need time and vision to order and shape our
lives. We struggle to understand our experiences and the people
around us. We attempt to make sense of ourselves and our
sometimes unmanageable parts, touching the chaos of our interior self and realizing that we may safely befriend it.

Maturity finally comes with the washing away of all that
holds us back or impedes our healing and our progress toward
becoming our ultimate selves. Maturity explores the possibilities. It touches our humanness with compassion. It wrestles
with only the real things that obstruct our path to a life of gratitude. Maturity means celebrating the memory of our past and
preserving the wisdom that the past gives to today and to the
new ordering of our lives. Finally, the acceptance that comes
with maturity signals a breakthrough in that it releases us from
our enclosures and teaches us how to love.

CHAPTER 22

Gardens as a Source
of Healing

❧

*Every person harbors within himself or herself the artist's
vocation to create, whether that be expressed in one's love
for cooking or sewing, for dancing or loving, for storytelling or mechanical repairing. To encourage the artist
in another is to create a spirit-filled community.*

—Matthew Fox, *On Becoming a Musical,
Mystical Bear*

HER MOTHER DIED in July. Kate described herself as an orphan.

Shortly before her mother's death, a friend wrote to Kate sharing his own feelings upon the death of his second parent.

"The most distressing part for me," explained the friend,
"was the fact that my father's death set off an inescapable chain
of events. First, there was the process of sorting through a house
indelibly marked by my parents' pastimes and personal effects.
Plaid flannel shirts worn thin from years of predawn barn chores.
Canceled checks written to the local co-op equity. A dog-eared
address book containing every one of my telephone numbers since
my graduation from college. A calendar with a picture of their
local bank. Something in the depth of me trembled with loneliness
as I worked my way through everything from a grease-stained

135

apple dumpling recipe to church directory photos and appointment books. In a matter of hours I had taken an entire tour of their daily route, a chapter of my history that now needed to be put to rest. There I sat, reviewing the plain threads and simple stitches that basted together the whole of my parents' marriage. I was, at once, moved by and envious of their uncomplicated life together. Their time together spoke of a simplicity I had misplaced many years before. Never have I felt so alone and small."

Kate continued to relate the friend's story. "We then held the classic farm auction to disperse of my father's treasured tools and machinery . . . a herd of dairy cattle and several tons of hay. Finally, we had to let go of our family farm. We said good-bye to our cherished home, which had been a safe haven of predictability that welcomed us back whenever the world felt too hostile or strange. I felt as if I had been cut loose from my moorings. Set adrift. Even strangely free. While I can accept the fact that my future will be appreciably different without my parents, I sense that everything is now headed down an uncharted road, and I'm supposed to be adult enough to direct the course. More frightening, I can already tell this is a path I must make myself . . . by walking it."

Kate then spoke of her similar reaction to the loss of her mother in July. The death clearly struck many complex emotional chords in her heart. At the age of forty-eight, Kate found herself revisiting everything from her own life choices to her lack of plans for aging and caring for herself. Her dreams, won and lost, appeared in startling detail before her eyes. The richness of a superb education and a fine career contrasted with her feelings of inadequacy about her failed marriage. The joys of lasting friendships and two thriving children were tempered by the frustrations of her own chronic illness. The days and weeks all of a sudden seemed much more complicated for her when she faced them as a team of one. Suddenly she felt compelled to tell her mother's story, perhaps in search of clues to her own future.

"Her life and death bore much evidence of holiness," Kate explained. "Beyond her obvious goodness, her unconditional support of my brother and me and her splendidly gentle disposition, she grasped an essential truth about the meaning of 'holy.' She enacted this through her music, her friendships, and even in the pragmatic silliness that inspired her discipline of us children. She confirmed it daily through unpretentious fun marked by picnics, nasturtiums, needlework, Greek history, gin rummy, and fly-fishing. She was, to put it simply, an icon of hospitality and purveyor of good food. I never remember not wanting to see my mother," Kate added wistfully.

"For as long as I can remember, my mother loved to drive through the countryside tracking down mushrooms and wildflowers and teaching us how to identify them. With a bucket of water planted on the floor of the car, we would set out along the Chippewa River through Druand, Eau Galle, Ellsworth, and Spring Valley, Wisconsin. All the while she would offer a running commentary on everything from bird migrations to bouncing bett, monarch butterflies, fireweed, and poocoon. At least once during the drive she would remind us that it was impossible to see anything good from inside the car.

"Maybe it was her instinctive ability to look beyond the obvious for beauty. All I know is, whenever we scrambled out of the car for one of her enforced nature walks, we witnessed a fascinating world. And, as she predicted, none of it was visible from the road. My mother really had a gift for raising up those roadside treasures to a place of veneration. She knew how to exalt the small stuff."

Years earlier, during the Great Depression, Kate's mother had learned that to celebrate life together was to appreciate its mix of hues and moods. She knew what it meant to be present to the daily *experience of those she cared about. She truly enjoyed the beauty of creation and the essential goodness of life.*

It occurred to me as Kate spoke how often we construct mountains of obstacles fortified by heaps of "should"s and "must"s that prevent us from being where our hearts want to be. How easy it is to get caught up in the battle for survival, the hectic and pressured tasks that define our days. How easy it is to say, "If only I could do this, or mend that relationship, or earn more money, or travel—then I could finally relax and begin to appreciate my life." Actually, most of us probably don't need to change one thing in our lives to find an excuse to rejoice. We don't have to do big things, only small things well.

Shortly after telling me this story, Kate reported that she had gone to her mother's garden and begun to dig with a spade she'd retrieved from her parents' home. She dug phlox and daylilies. She found some nodding trillium and even a jack-in-the-pulpit. She described digging everything that looked as if it might like to live in her garden.

Next she decided to call some close friends to see if they had plants she might have. This produced several fancy irises, a white peony, and a rosebush. Kate continued her little quest until she had dug up much of her yard and fashioned several new flower beds. She then labeled each plant, took photographs of them as they bloomed, and produced a small sketchbook filled with pictures, poems, and notes about each person who had given her a plant. The garden became for her a living commentary on friendships and love. And in the center of all this resided her mother's wildflowers and famous "Magic" lilies. Kate's creative insights were glorious and clearly helped her address issues of loss. To create, for her, was to be freed from emotional and physical pain.

CARING FOR MYSELF AND OTHERS

Some people seem to have a natural instinct for looking after their own souls, especially at critical crossroads in their lives. Women like Kate, for example, tend to reflect honestly on their place in the world and then determine a healing course of action. For the rest of us, and for those who watch and worry about friends and loved ones who don't seem to know how to care for themselves spiritually, emotionally, or even physically, the following suggestions may help.

Matters in need of attention include

> My mental and emotional health
> Care of my body and physical self
> Learning and growing intellectually
> Nourishing my spiritual self
> Valuing humor
> Attending to my creative self
> Building and preserving important relationships in my life

With respect to each, ask yourself three questions: Where am I now? What could I do to improve my spiritual health? What *will* I do?

"Today," said Kate, "when I drive along the country roads of my childhood, I realize that a part of my mother still lives with me in my garden. And July, the month of her death, is a good month to begin the feast. With its soil-rich fields of grain and verdant woodlands, its telephone lines festooned with meadowlarks and mourning doves, July is the growing season of life in the human heart and in the soil of creation. It is a time when the earth sends up new grass as it puts down deep roots."

July, for Kate, has become a spiritual moment and a doorway to the future—albeit a future changed by the passing of someone she loved. But she has turned the corner on another winter, slogged her way through a muddy spring, and now plans to take a chance once more to step with faith into a future of prospects. July is a month when her thoughts always return to her garden and home, to her mother.

History and tradition matter a great deal. For example, the Anglican tradition, in which I grew up, embraces a theology that underscores the earthly presence of God. Signs of this closeness brush our consciousness through countless things, including magnificent cathedrals and other holy architecture. Music, liturgy, poetry, stained glass, and gardens also fall within the promise of God's active presence in the world. In its own way, each expression of beauty enhances our experience of creation and a higher power. Each helps to shape a world of such awe that we cannot resist "falling in love with God."

In my experience, those who, like Kate, believe the world is basically a beautiful place—even if it came about because of nature rather than because of God—have a reason to remain in it. A person who believes in a benevolent source of creation has a potent reason for hope, and hope means everything when it comes to being well.

CHAPTER 23

The Role of Spiritual Development in Health

❧❦

THE TERM "MODERNITY" can refer to an intellectual ideology that began with the French Revolution. Its basic constructs of optimism, scientific humanism, narcissistic hedonism, reductionism, and individualism have marked our culture in ways that have not necessarily fostered good health. In fact, these principles have failed to produce the abundant and suffering-free life they originally promised, giving rise instead to a sense of malaise and a longing for spiritual roots. We as a nation have become painfully aware that suffering and pain are a permanent part of the fabric of the human condition. Any victory we've achieved over either has been only temporary and elusive.[1]

The spiritual aspects of life involve the ways in which we live our beliefs each day. At the level of spirit is where we find strength and identity and an energy that comes from something beyond our self. At the level of spirit, we also sense a source of wisdom and order, a truth that can be trusted even as life changes and we encounter a world of disorder. Spiritual qualities tend to surface when we discover that making our body and mind feel good isn't enough and sometimes isn't even possible. Spiritual assets grow as we find ourselves walking a new and unexpected path, or face an unplanned hurdle.

A whole person seeks the joy of living at the level of spirit. More and more, as we grow older and mature, this joy begins to outshine the pleasures we once used to comfort our bodies and minds. We see that the ideals embodied in modernity, the overemphasis on individual autonomy, and the materialistic goals we might have set out for ourselves lack both substance and durability. We realize with increasing certainty that the relationship between physical well-being and spiritual vitality is intricate and real.[2]

At any time, no matter how bad things have become or how dire the consequences of disease, loss, or injury, it is also possible to attain wholeness. With or without a cure, this kind of wholeness happens at the level of spirit and is marked by attention to narrative and to relationships. Living in the realm of spirit offers each of us the potential for new beginnings—a chance to see life through the eyes of our souls and to listen with the ears of our hearts.

CHAPTER 24

The Power of Story

⋗⋖

Lord, hear my voice: let thine ears be attentive to the voice of my supplications.

—Psalm 130

COMPASSION CELEBRATES *as well as acts mercifully. To live out compassion requires that we listen. Compassion, like love and justice, is an act of creation. All three engender health, and all three begin with listening.*

The expression on Dorothy's face said it all. Her anguish over a grim cancer prognosis reached beyond the limits of any religious argument or emotional preparation. As I gazed upon her devastated countenance and ashen complexion, I remembered—again— the fear and vulnerability that accompany serious illness. No textbook or set of guiding principles prepares us to fully respond to this kind of panic. Though intellectualizing pain is often a first line of defense, sometimes it's important to let pain be pain, erring on the side of silence rather than getting caught up in platitudes or unhelpful theological assertions.

"I'm seventy-six years old," Dorothy explained with enormous effort. "I thought that this was just the way you feel when you get to be seventy-six."

In fact, Dorothy had not felt well for at least a year. Several visits to her local physician had led to no answers about her failing health. Maybe her problem was depression. Perhaps she needed vitamins or some iron to prop up her sinking body. In any case, it hardly mattered now. Yesterday's surgery had revealed enough about her metastasized stomach cancer to make clear that she needed to get her life in order. If that wasn't bad enough news, her doctor chose to break his grim report to a roomful of Dorothy's unsuspecting family members, including several very young grandchildren.

"The doctor never even shared a word of this with me first," reported Dorothy sadly. *"I had no idea how serious the cancer was. I'll never get over the expressions of terror on my children's faces. The way he talked, I felt more like a medical chart than a person."*

All the while, according to Dorothy, the doctor acted impatient to get on with his day. He leaned lightly against the door frame, drumming his fingertips, seemingly anxious to extract himself from this inconvenience. In a matter of about eight minutes, he had dismissed nearly eight decades of her life, treating her as if she were nothing more than a diagnostic mistake. What he might have called professional detachment felt to her like a personal insult from a faceless mechanic.

That had all taken place the day before. Today, with family and physician absent, Dorothy and I sat together in her room. A construction crew pounded and shoveled concrete outside her window, oblivious to the news that a woman's life would be ending soon.

"Tell me about your children," I asked.

Dorothy looked surprised at being asked something that had nothing to do with cancer. *"We had eleven children—five boys and six girls,"* she reported. *"One of the girls died in a car accident on the night of her prom. Let's see, that was 1969. Kathleen, my daughter, had the prettiest blond hair and blue eyes, just like my husband. You probably read about it in the paper. That was a bad year for kids getting into car accidents around our place."*

I had not read about Kathleen's accident but did remember a spate of car crashes during the mid-sixties. Several teens near my own home had died.

Dorothy's had been a rural life, the life of a dairy farmer's mate, a mother who baked fourteen loaves of bread a week and packed as many as seven school lunches every day. She came from a small town tucked in a valley near the St. Croix River.

"One year I canned over a thousand quarts of fruits and vegetables," she offered with increasing brightness. "I guess it was everything from green beans to applesauce. Of course, that didn't include the rolls, cookies, and pies that went through my kitchen every week. I was a real good cook, but you know, I never even had time to learn to drive until my youngest went off to school. Finally one day, after all the kids were out of the house, I put out some bales of straw and learned how to parallel park the car. Passed the driver's test too . . . the very first time. I was over forty before I ever got behind the wheel, except for a tractor now and then.

"After that I took some time for myself. I signed up for a ceramics class in town and had a little fun. We used to play cards some with the neighbors. The kids all played in the band and sang in the choir. Only a couple of the boys played ball, but that was because they had a lot of chores to take care of here at home. They all live nearby now. Nice children. Respectful and such. I have sixty grandchildren, don't you know.

"And my mother, well she lived about ten miles away, over there near Plum City. She used to have a good old time playing canasta with her friends every week. By the way, you didn't ever know a Vivian Holmstead, did you? She was my mother's best friend. Finally Mother got too crippled up with arthritis to plant her own garden, so I'd go down to her place and do it for her. She'd watch from the screen porch and say to me, 'Now, Dorothy, that's just the way I would plant it. You always did know how to

do things right, like planting the marigolds around the edges to keep the rabbits out of the garden.'

"Then Mother would make me lunch and tell me how I never eat enough. It was usually BLTs or lettuce and onions from her garden wilted with fried bacon and a little vinegar. There's nothin' better, in my book."

"Now that your life has taken a different turn, how do you think you and your family will manage?" I asked.

"Well, I don't know about my husband. He's not real handy around the house. He's retired, you know, but he still helps our son farm, just to keep himself busy. When he's home, he sticks pretty close to the family room with his TV and snacks. At eighty-one, I just don't know how much help he could be. Maybe he could cook a little, or pick things up at the deli in town. I'll have to say though, he sure surprised me when he brought these pretty little pearl earrings. 'I looked for a dainty pair,' he says to me, 'just the way you always liked them.' Maybe he could do a few more things if I let him."

"I think you're right, Dorothy. He might even like doing a few more things," I replied.

Dorothy talked for a long time that afternoon, much longer than I would have expected for someone as frail as she appeared. She actually seemed to gain energy with each new topic. Intuitively, through our review of her life, she reconstructed personal memories with a sense that life had been worthwhile. Her process was one that let her take ownership of her individual history and find renewed satisfaction in her choices. Unfortunately for her physician, he missed that entire experience.

"The people who come to see us bring us their stories," says the psychiatrist and writer Robert Coles. "They hope they tell them well enough so that we understand the truth of their lives."

A physician who learned the power of story early in his training, Coles attaches great value to the accumulated stories in our lives. No one's stories are quite like anyone else's, and doctors need to become diggers, trying hard to follow treasure maps in hopes of discovering gold.[1]

Anytime we invite someone else to share a life story, we are saying that she is valuable and her history is significant. Since the story that grows from one's past also contributes to the shape of the present, telling it is a valuable exercise. Life reviews have been especially helpful for bereavement counselors who support families and dying patients. They also provide fruitful invitations to elderly friends or patients. Through having conversations and examining family photos and letters, an individual can assimilate and integrate all kinds of things that must be addressed before he or she can say good-bye. Others, like Dorothy, benefit in simply knowing that their lives haven't been wasted, that it has all been worthwhile in the end. Still others find that this review gives them a starting point from which they can begin afresh.

Pastoral counseling involves a kind of counseling that helps guide the inner life of others as they walk through a crisis. This includes helping someone such as Dorothy articulate her own stories in an effort toward closure. This is especially true when the medical situation offers little or no promise of cure.

Taking care of someone's soul consists of engaging that person in conversation focused on her or his well-being. It points someone toward the healing process, which, unlike curing, engenders integration of what used to be and what is now. The fact remains that scientific knowledge alone does not fix or even help this kind of situation. Everyone involved—and that includes Dorothy's doctor—needs something stronger to hold on to. Everyone needs to recognize that meaning is as valuable as knowledge, and that meaning can change the experience of illness in profound ways—for both doctor and patient. This kind of change happens at the level of soul.

Taking care of someone's soul also can involve ritual. This might encompass anything from praying to lighting votive

LIFE AS A NARRATIVE WORTH SHARING

At some point along the way I began to realize that life is not just a journey but a narrative—a winding trail of words and symbols from childhood to maturity, and from youth to age; from innocence to awareness, and from ignorance to knowing; from foolishness to discretion, and then, perhaps, to wisdom; from weakness to strength, or from strength to weakness; from health to sickness, and back, we pray, to health; from offense to forgiveness; from loneliness to love; from joy to gratitude; from pain to compassion, and from grief to understanding; from fear to faith; from defeat to reconciliation . . . until, looking backward or ahead, we finally see that victory lies not at some high place along the way, but in having made the journey stage by stage.

candles. Anointing, blessing, remembering, and storytelling also constitute spiritually satisfying activities to share with someone like Dorothy. And it doesn't take a chaplain to accompany someone on this healing journey.

In short, when we aim toward restoring whole persons, we offer a perspective based on concern and solicitude for whole persons. We encourage people to look at their lives as part of a greater story. If the medical world has been accused of dealing with patients in a compartmentalized, hyperrational way, it's because certain health professionals have lost sight of the broader and more subjective aspects of health. In reality, each of us, whether physician or friend, can bring to another the promise that life, even a life altered by disease or injury, has meaning and value. It is a gift to be celebrated and cherished, one that needs to be remembered through personal story.

We live in difficult times for the health care world. Who we are and what impact we have as medical and spiritual caregivers depends largely on our personal courage. Do we have the courage to place ourselves in the midst of human suffering? Do we have the stamina to challenge those in the health care business world who say that suffering costs too much? There is certainly no shortage of misery.

To accompany another in pain is to enter into a relationship with that person. This relationship invites us to serve life rather than fix life. It speaks to the issue of connecting with another rather than performing with competence. This is the place where both believers and nonbelievers recognize that God is present. If we aim only to fix disease, without restoring whole persons, we miss the core meaning of health. If we have neither the time nor the inclination to be in relationship with others, we miss all those awe-inspiring situations in which we can partake of a holy presence with those who may have no hope. And isn't it hope that we are ultimately called to bring to others?

CHAPTER 25

Cultivating the Art of Being

❧❦

*If they get nothing else, I hope my students get these things
from me: You have to love medicine or leave it. Every day
you're a learner. Every day you're a listener. You will never
go wrong if you treat your patient as a family member.
Practicing medicine is not a job, it's an honor.*

> —Matthew Segedy, M.D.,
> chief pediatric resident,
> St. Paul Children's Hospital

ONE DAY *a group of medical residents asked how they might
remain a support to a family whose child showed few signs of getting better; they had done all they could do medically. The little
girl had come to the hospital nearly a month earlier with a multi-
tude of problems, including unmanageable seizures, followed by a
difficult surgery and a long, slow process of waking up. Persistent
infections and a host of other complications suggested that this little girl might not ever fully awaken and might not even leave the
hospital. Each day medical and other staff expressed more anxiety
at not knowing how to interact with the family, especially when
they knew little about the child's prognosis.*

*The residents, in particular, expressed this concern. On the one
hand, they wanted to stay connected with the little girl's parents.*

151

*On the other hand, they felt awkward about having no helpful
medical information to offer. Their awkwardness combined with
their lack of authority made it difficult for them to walk into a
room full of anguished family members. Such an endeavor clearly
called for skills that their training or professional experience had
not taught them so far.*

*After talking about some possibilities, we concluded that the
first thing they might have to do upon entering the child's room
was simply to take a deep breath, sit down, and count to ten. Once
they quelled their urge to jump up and leave, they might begin a
conversation by telling the family how sorry they were about their
child's ongoing health crisis. Acknowledging the parents' courage
during this difficult time could also help establish a movement
toward empathy and conversation. The residents might also consider telling the parents how powerless they felt at having so little
clear medical information to offer them about their child's future.*

*Once they reached some small point of confidence, they could
ask a parent or other family member to tell them all the reasons
they loved this little girl. What was she like? What did she bring
to their lives? What did they enjoy doing together? The residents
decided they would encourage the parents to bring in family photos
and personal items to help hospital staff get to know their daughter, as they knew her. Last, though maybe most important, the residents would work at becoming comfortable with sitting in silence
or listening to another's frustration without attempting to fix it.*

When suffering and worry spill over into words, the one thing
bereaved people need is someone to listen without judgment. If
the suffering person is exhausted or doesn't feel like talking, it's
wise to accept the silence, which is far better than aimless chatter. Many times, our presence is exactly what someone needs,
even if this presence involves very few words.

Unfortunately, our current model of practicing medicine
sometimes treats presence without action as an expression of

utter inadequacy. Actually, our entire culture reacts similarly. To those whose lives consist of performing an enormous list of tasks, presence without action means wasted time and money. It smacks of diminished quality and squandered resources, medical and human. Because presence cannot be measured or managed, it's hard for some people to take it very seriously. Yet, being present to those who are ill, and paying attention to their souls, could prove to be one of the most important aspects of health care.

"We cannot really experience anything without being present to it," says the psychotherapist and writer Gunilla Norris. "True presence requires that we be attentive to what is happening . . . here and now. It is an offering of our awareness, our participation, and our willingness. This is a basic and profound courtesy. By such courtesy we are deeply transformed."[1]

A chaplain's experience contradicts the notion that offering our presence is simply a nice thing to do. Maybe it's because we see that those who are ill and dying need the presence of a community of friends, family, and health care providers for support and fellowship, not just for a cure. Or maybe we realize that the community of friends and caregivers needs the presence of the dying to make them think about eternal issues—to make them listen. A hospital furnishes a wonderful snapshot of the life-giving potential within a vocation of presence.

By their nature, serious illness and death invite us to become reflective, to put down our masks and begin that inward journey in search of what is ultimately worthy and good about life. The prospect of death nudges both patients and their companions toward their own mortality. It bids them to ask who they are and where they stand with their relationships and commitments. How do they give life to others? Where do they find God's creative presence in their lives? The prospect of death calls each of us to consider these questions.

Anytime we find ourselves standing in the reality of human suffering, we find it is a humbling experience. Suffering involves real people who find precious little comfort in philosophic argument or scriptural interpretation. We dare not intellectualize the meaning of another's suffering, for it cannot be reduced to rational answers. We also must not avoid the meaning of suffering, as we then avoid a significant piece of life, including our own life.

Instead, we're wise to let the wondering that has haunted humankind from the beginning become our wondering. Why is there needless suffering in the world? Why do innocent children die? Where is the God of love and compassion in our time of need? Families always wonder about this. Patients, including children, wonder as well. These questions are as old as human memory and point to a twofold task we face in our search to be well.

First, we must ask ourselves how we personally reconcile ourselves to, or how do we reconcile suffering with a loving God? How do we feel about death and can we accept that some things defy fixing? Some situations will never see much improvement, though nearly all situations can find transformation. Once we accept the fact that there is no satisfactory or rational explanation for human suffering, we give up the idea of finding an intellectual solution and start looking for creative, generative ways of responding to the presence of sorrow and its consequences.

The trouble with all this is that today's approach to health and health care does not encourage relationship or presence as ways of treating disease. Health care providers boldly do many things to patients. They poke and prod. They test and measure and rule out, sometimes missing the large picture. They learn early in their careers to avoid asking patients open-ended questions, for fear the patients might use up precious reimbursement money with long-winded (though eminently valuable) answers. They discover that they must see far too many patients in an hour or a day to justify sitting around with any one. Those who

Illness and the Inner Life

"If the focus of the 20th century has been on outer space, the focus of the 21st century may well be on inner space. We are entering a new era of discovery—not of the world around us, but of the world within. The disappointments of the external world; the headlong pursuit of hedonism and materialism; and the callous disregard of people for each other—all have driven people to look within themselves for ways to understand and deal with life. There are clear signs that people in all societies have an intense hunger for healing of mind, body and soul," said George Gallup, Jr., chairman, Gallup International Institute, at a December 1998 presentation he made at Harvard's spirituality and healing conference.

For the past thirty years:

Ninety-five percent of Americans say they believe in God.
Eighty percent of people surveyed considered religion to be "important" or "very important."
Among people over sixty-five, 85 percent agreed that "my religious faith is the most important influence on my life."
In a study of elderly patients, 78 percent of the respondents stated that they would appreciate their personal physician praying with them during times of great physical or emotional crisis.[2]

Religious and other spiritual factors continue to be neglected in the practice of medicine, even though patients and families feel they're important and wish to address them. Whether one is coping with loneliness or trying to live fully with a chronic illness, the health of the inner life must find its way back into medical practice. Without soul care, people cannot hope to find a sense of peace and well-being.

begin their medical training espousing lofty ideals and pristine practice standards eventually learn that, upon joining a medical practice, they may have to see a patient every seven to eight minutes.

Meanwhile, the medical residents who were searching for ways to relate to the little girl's family learned their lesson well. Several times following our discussion, I passed the child's room and eventually saw each of the residents, one by one, sitting comfortably with the family. The mother later said to me that she had never seen so many conscientious young physicians who took such a genuine interest in her child. This seemingly hopeless situation, while producing little medical progress, became a source of trust and sustenance for everyone involved.

Thomas Aquinas once said: "The truly reasonable is the truly good." For anyone who embraces a genuine interest in wholeness, a vocation of presence embodies both the reasonable and the good. Further, I am convinced that the lack of these aspects of human relationship has the potential to kill both the art of medicine and the whole of our culture.

HOPE   *Trust or reliance; desire accompanied by expectancy; an expectation of future good. Hope is larger and more courageous than wishes. Unlike a specific set of expectations that attempt to put certain limitations on life, hope believes that life can emerge from even the most difficult of circumstances. Hope defies all boundaries and refuses to accept misery as an option. Hope is a gift we can bring to others who are ill or struggling with loss and discouragement.*

CHAPTER 26

The Importance of Nurturing Children's Spiritual Life as Well as Our Own

❦

IF CARE OF SOUL has important effects on our health and the health of those we love, it has even more critical implications for the lives of children. Helping children develop inner resources—character, positive attitudes, problem-solving skills, acceptance of others, coping, and a sense of humor—helps prepare them for life in general, including life's losses and illness. Being present and paying attention create the foundation for nurturing children's spiritual development. Having fun together can take that development to a higher level.

My son's tenth birthday served as the backdrop for a lesson in youthful spiritual development and silliness, particularly with respect to gender competencies and roles.

Christian invited several boys from his sixth-grade class to spend the day and night at our farm. None of them was acquainted with rural life, and Prairie View Farm had much entertainment to offer. The boys arrived about noon and, following my brief speech about farm rules, disappeared for most of the afternoon. I caught only an occasional glimpse of them running behind the house and through the pasture, or huddled in the machine shed kicking tractor tires. At one point, Christian shouted at me to come see how they had managed to slip a halter on our orphan Hereford calf, Ben. Ben was both stout and precocious. Clearly delighted with all the attention, he returned the favor by dragging the young cowboys behind him around the calf pen. This comical little rodeo caused quite a stir among the adult cattle, and they responded by galloping in circles, tossing their tails high in the air. Fortunately the livestock executed these maneuvers on the other side of the fence. Even our bull, Halsey, left his charges and ambled over to the gate for a better look. It was a raucous mix of boys, bulls, tractors, and mud—a solid stage for a day of formative masculine seasoning.

Several hours later I met the birthday guests swaggering up the driveway toward the house, seemingly much more robust and self-confident than they had been a few hours earlier. Hungry and exhausted, their knees caked with cow manure, the boys radiated youthful virility. One could only imagine their parents' expressions of astonishment when they heard about the day's exploits on the farm.

Then, as the group came within shouting distance I heard, "Mom, get your shotgun." Christian apparently had one more manly demonstration he wished to share with his friends.

"What on earth for?" I called back with matching vigor.

"These guys want to see you shoot your gun," he replied, giving the boys a self-assured glance. "I told them you really knew how to shoot, and you could probably hit practically anything."

It certainly wasn't a very politically correct request, though it did rather match the day's level of bravado. I tried to redirect their interest toward something a little more birthdaylike, such as the homemade pizza waiting for them in the kitchen. I might as well have asked them to clean the house. Christian had already

informed his friends that in a locked cabinet I kept an old
Winchester Model 12 shotgun that had belonged to my mother.
Captured by the idea that I might even know how to shoot it, they
all nudged one another, begging Christian to apply some pressure
on Mother. This was not going to be easy.

After failing to change anybody's mind, I finally gave in. At
least it would be an opportunity to give them a little lesson in gun
safety. I went to the house, removed my gun from the cabinet, and
selected a single shell from the box before rejoining the expectant
audience waiting in the driveway. Maybe I could just shoot up in
the air or over our woods. The noise alone would probably sat-
isfy them.

"What do you want me to shoot?" I asked the sports fans.
"There's nothing much around here except trees and alfalfa."
In unison, they all looked skyward, scanning the horizon for
a possible target.

"There!" shouted Christian. "Get that bird up there. Mom,
you can hit it, I know you can. Just try it. Hurry before it gets
away. Hurry."

The late-afternoon sky revealed nothing more than an
approaching sunset. Fortunately, as far as the human eye could
see there were no unsuspecting crows, no roosting pigeons, no
hawks hunting for field mice. I couldn't see a single thing—with
the exception of one small black speck that looked to be a mid-
sized cricket flying a very safe distance away. For that matter, it
could have been a barn swallow in the next county. In either case,
any self-respecting hunter would have known she could never hit
it from where we stood. Assured that I would miss my target, I
brought the gun to my shoulder, aimed into the air vaguely in the
direction of the swooping speck, and fired.

Every cow in the pasture swung its head up and gawked
curiously. Even Halsey looked appropriately impressed. Nothing
approaching logic could have explained why I hit that bird from
such a distance. Obviously it was a fluke. Every reasonable

HEALTHY CHILDREN NEED HEALTHY SOULS

Strong, healthy, prospering children are not simply born that way. They must be nourished with the essentials of good health and development. "Developmental assets," according to the Search Institute of Minneapolis, Minnesota, are more than nice ideas that we all agree can help children. They provide the mortar that holds together a foundation upon which young people can shape their lives. The forty developmental assets identified by the Search Institute show a dramatic correlation with the choices young people make. The more assets young people have, the less likely they are to engage in problem behaviors and activities that threaten their overall health. Assets help protect youth from high-risk behaviors such as alcohol and tobacco use, abuse of marijuana and other drugs, sexual activity, violence, and attempted suicide.

Developmental assets do more than protect against risky, health-compromising behaviors. They also promote school success, the affirmation of diversity, and good social behavior. Research such as the Search Institute's indicates that increasing young people's experiences of assets can not only reduce problems involving youth but also enlarge young people's contribution to the community, now and in the future.

calculation would have favored the bird, yet, amazingly it dropped from the sky like a rock. We all gazed skyward in giddy amazement. The boys exchanged disbelieving glances, first at one another, then at me. They charged off wildly to retrieve the small feathered booty, delivering it back to the house for my inspection. It was a low moment in the life of a once-competent trap shooter.

From that day forward, however, I enjoyed a new level of distinction among the local sixth-grade boys. Word soon got out that

Since 1990, the Search Institute has identified a forty-asset framework of internal and external resources that all children need to grow up healthy, competent, and caring. Extensive research led Search Institute to identify the essential building blocks of adolescent development. These building blocks include twenty external assets and twenty internal assets. External assets fall into four categories: support, empowerment, boundaries and expectations, and constructive use of time. Some of the nurturing benefits that fall within these primary categories are family support, other adult relationships, service to others, family and school boundaries, creative activities, and youth programs.

The four primary categories of internal assets include commitment to learning, positive values, social competencies, and positive identity. Some qualities that fall within these categories are commitment to learning, integrity and honesty, planning and decision making, interpersonal competence, resistance skills, peaceful conflict resolution, personal power, and sense of purpose. To learn more about research surrounding healthy youth, contact the Search Institute at 700 S. Third Street, Suite 210, Minneapolis, MN 55415-1138 (www.search-institute.org).

I could take down a bird from at least a mile, maybe five. Overnight, I became the star sportswoman of the PTA set. Several parents and at least one teacher inquired about the extraordinary event. Young boys started calling the house and asking for me, as if I had won a gold medal in the pentathlon. The coming school year, Christian and several members of his traveling hockey team asked if I would like to be their coach. All in all, it became a high point in oddball parenting heroics.

For me, the sharpshooting caper demonstrated some aspects of soul formation and spiritual health in children. First, I believe that most of us underestimate the degree to which we influence children—our own and others'. Whether we care for their physical health, pack their lunches, or teach second grade, we have as many rich opportunities to shape their hearts and spirits as we do to mold their minds and bodies. Second, unlike brown eyes and blond hair, sexism, violence, and prejudice do not come naturally to children. Young people, in my experience, view life much more holistically. What this really says is that all of us who interact with young people, all of us who help shape their lives in meaningful ways, who teach children, encourage them, protect their health, and nurture them, must approach our tasks as both awesome privilege and immense responsibility.

CHAPTER 27

Doubt and Questioning Can Shed Light on Meaning

❧❧

It seems that each passing year brings more clutter and activity into my space. Without question, silence and solitude play a more important role, as they have become sources of nourishment for me. Yet, spending time with people who struggle with health issues tells me that, during times of pain or questioning or in seasons of doubt, we can easily become dangerous weapons against ourselves—especially if we choose to spend too much time alone. Isolation, like heresy, begins with a thread of truth and stretches it into an unrecognizable lie. It can become a priceless treasure turned to poison. In fact, individuals recovering from alcoholism have said that, every time they feel the need to isolate themselves from others, they know that what they really want is a drink. There is a fine line between solitude and isolation.

Isolation invites self-absorption and self-centeredness. When we set out to get away from those who bother us or make our lives complicated, we lose our objectivity. We convince ourselves of untruths, get our priorities mixed up, and, in the words of my wonderfully astute father, "attempt to fool a damn good person."

I suspect that one reason we sometimes avoid the community of others is that we are afraid someone might tell us something we suspect is true but would rather deny. Community, after all, consists of a body of shared truths. That body of truths has a unique way of maintaining a more genuine honesty than any individual assertions of truth can possibly attain.

The relationship between helplessness and doubt is much like that between isolation and solitude. While unattended helplessness can lead to gratuitous self-pity or stuck-in-the-mire imprisonment, doubt involves movement. It implies that something will eventually be resolved.

Indeed, doubt's most vital function is that it compels us to find answers. Doubt ultimately demands the truth. When in doubt, one cannot simply flounder about indefinitely without taking any kind of action. One needs only to look at the development of our whole technical civilization since the time of the Enlightenment. It has been built on doubt. Enormous achievements in medicine have come about because someone doubted someone else's previous methods. Doubt has pushed us forward into vast new frontiers of knowledge.

Think of the discoveries and events of recent history that are founded in doubt. We have come to doubt the viability of nuclear war. We doubt that our earth can hold up much longer under the ecological siege we have put to her. We doubt that business and industry know how to responsibly look after the environment. We doubt that assault rifles are a necessary commodity for hunters or that blind faith in any government is a sound idea. Some of us doubt the wisdom of aggressive medical intervention and treatment at any cost.

These kinds of doubts can actually lead us to a kind of conversion. They turn us around and invite us to step up to a different level of truth. By pulling us toward a higher level of consciousness and maturity, they awaken new sensitivity. Good things can emerge from doubting, as was the case with a physician who developed colon cancer at the peak of an illustrious career in which he doubted much and discovered more:

A neonatologist who began caring for critically ill newborns when this field had just begun to emerge, Simon treated medicine as an adventure. He became a pioneer, working in a newborn intensive care unit with sick and prematurely born infants. At times he would retreat to the laboratory, where he searched for better techniques to treat tiny preemies with underdeveloped lungs. He lectured. He taught throughout the United States, Europe, and Japan. He enjoyed enormous success. He became a chronic doubter whose changes in treatment technology ultimately saved the lives of thousands of children.

Simon always had a clear view of who he was and what he wanted to accomplish as a physician. Patient care meant everything to him and, although he constantly dealt with lives in the balance, he maintained a remarkable sense of silliness and levity.

"There are people who care too much about the human condition and not enough about the Minnesota Twins," he announced on numerous occasions. "It's so easy to get caught up in the details and miss the drama."

He knew how to focus on what was important and, at the same time, enjoy other things around him. A man with strong opinions about patient care, Simon once found himself in the middle of an insurance company–hospital dispute concerning who was going to pay for what. It seemed that a hospitalized baby with chronic health problems was generating a large medical bill that the family's insurance company was not prepared to pay. Nobody knew if the baby could stay. Finally, at some crucial point in this discussion, Simon succinctly announced his sentiments to the squabbling parties:

"If he goes, I go."

The baby stayed.

A letter he once received from a sixth-grader he had treated years ago also produced a quick response. The letter began, "Hi, I don't know if anyone remembers me . . ."

Simon immediately wrote back: "We do remember you. You were a very small, very sick baby, one of the first patients to receive a new therapy. . . . Many people think doctors and nurses are different, that we don't feel the same things other people do. That's not really true . . . we are just ordinary people working in somewhat extraordinary jobs. Your letter reminded us of how wonderfully extraordinary our jobs really are."

The word "ecstasy" originates in the Greek *ekstasis*, which derives from *ek*, meaning out, and *stasis*, a state of standstill. In other words, to be ecstatic means to be outside of a fixed place. We can recognize people who live ecstatic lives because they are always moving away from static situations. They are the doubtful and restless explorers who always hunt for unmapped territory to investigate. An ecstatic person thrives on doubt, knowing that uncertainty and skepticism precede the discovery of truth.

Simon exemplified the ecstatic person, who lives in a place where determination constantly breaks through the walls of uncertainty. When he chose to live ecstatically, he chose a shared life, a life in community with others who also allowed themselves to doubt and learn with him. He left the safe, secure, familiar place of rigid medical beliefs and pat solutions and reached out to others as he cared for their sick and dying children. He boldly ventured onto untilled soil, even when it involved risking a journey into someone else's suffering. Ecstasy such as his always reaches out to new freedom—freedom from oppression, injustice, and ignorance.

Conversely, static living separates us and transforms us into self-absorbed individuals fighting for our own individual survival. Ecstatic living brings us together, to discover one another, to be responsible for one another, and to proclaim life as creative and filled with potential. At the center of this timeless and elementary philosophy lies the heart of an all-encompassing human family.

As Simon became increasingly ill, he often spoke about the meaning of his work. "I'm so happy to have had a job that made a difference," he would say. "How incredible it's been to be invited into people's lives at such critical junctures—to walk with them and know them. Sometimes people would come up and thank me for something I had done years ago, or tell me how well their child was doing. Sometimes students would do the same. You just never know when you could influence someone's life."

What did this restless, questioning, opinionated, politically incorrect, and dying medical adventurer want to tell young physicians about to begin practice? "Show up, listen, and tell the truth," Simon replied, without missing a beat. Even at the end of his life, curiosity drove his clinical research, while his sensitivity to patients and their families helped ease the pain of their anxious vigils.

Finally, in a voice edged with something between humility and doubt, he added,

"I did the best I could . . . at least, I think so."

CHAPTER 28

The Heart of Health

⊸🙣🙡⊷

Love and intimacy are at the root of what makes us sick and what makes us well, what causes sadness and what brings happiness, what makes us suffer and what leads to healing.

—Dean Ornish, M.D.

IT SEEMS IMPOSSIBLE to talk about the heart of health without first acknowledging the power of love and of relationships in preserving and restoring health. The heart specialist Dean Ornish, M.D., approaches the subject of love and health from the perspectives of both a clinical researcher and a physician.

"Research shows . . . that people who feel lonely, depressed and isolated have three to five times greater rates of premature death and disease from virtually all causes compared to people who have a sense of love, connection and community," says Ornish. "I don't know anything in medicine, including drugs and surgery, that has such a powerful impact on death and disease. Yet these are things that we generally don't learn about in our medical training and we don't value in our culture."[1]

It seems that modern health care practice environments and the people who work in them sometimes appear to confuse health care with health care management; the terms are used almost interchangeably. I often hear young physicians in training refer to reimbursement issues and health care management rules as if they were part of a diagnosis or treatment plan. In truth, they have little or nothing to do with caring. Health care management pertains to the business of medicine—the marketing and money aspects of health care services. But to take up health care as a professional pursuit implies that one has some sense of altruism or interest in another's health. Health care has always involved itself with preservation of health as well as with the fair distribution and accessibility of health care resources. To care in this capacity is to advocate for and protect another, including a fragile or disenfranchised other. Caring involves assuming some level of responsibility for humankind. It is open to connecting with and listening to others.

"Many people have nowhere where they feel known, where they feel seen and heard and understood—and not just their good parts, but all of them—where people know their dark side, but they are still there for them, they still love them," relates Dr. Ornish.

How do we love others, particularly within the context of health? I have never been convinced that love is a *feeling*. Though it might elicit an emotion, love falls short of completion without an accompanying action. Genuine love implies responsibility and the exercise of wisdom. It encompasses a will to extend oneself—a vocation attended by consistent, predictable acts—not a sentiment. Love does not mean boundless giving; it means judicious giving and judicious withholding. Praising. Challenging. Arguing. Struggling. Confronting. Urging. Lifting up. Letting go. A judicious act requires leadership and wisdom, so love implies both.

Few things spoil love more quickly than dependency. Dependency cares little about personal or spiritual growth. When we are dependent, we care only about our own nourishment. We are not willing to tolerate any unhappiness or discomfort that accompanies growing in love. When we depend on another person for our own happiness or fulfillment, we have no wish to help that person grow, nor can we validate ourselves without that person.

Dependency implies smothering another by losing sight of the boundaries that keep one person from absorbing or sliding into another. Dependency invites such statements as "But I need her" and "Life means nothing without him." The same dependency that says, "I cannot go on without another," also fuels anxiety, depression, and unwholesome substitutes for genuine spiritual health.

I might fully adore another person's companionship. I might love someone deeply. I can touch and be touched by another. I might connect to another in ways that defy earthly description. But the day I need someone to ensure that my life is fruitful and productive, the day I demand that another person take charge of my emotional wholeness . . . that is the day when I have chosen something other than love or health.

Human sexuality is an energy that finds expression in the desire for contact, warmth, tenderness, and love. Sexuality further provides the motivation that fuels our search for intimacy or our encounter of being in touch. In the center of this search lie freedom and responsibility, in creative tension. Freedom without responsibility and commitment produces totally autonomous humans who wish to please only themselves. Blind commitment to another offers no tools for people to become whole. It says that there is no need to know oneself emotionally or spiritually.

If I do not know who I am, how can I share myself with a loved one? Some of the depth of me may be bright and creative. Some of me could be mysterious and untrustworthy. Part of me radiates strength and integrity. Other parts need repair and guidance. When all my parts work well together, I function as a harmonious whole, a more complete self who celebrates and shares in love with others. When I ignore myself and live through others, for others, or in anticipation of others feeding me, I have neglected to create conditions by which I can reach my full human potential. For, in order for me to know and love others, I must first know and love myself.

Loving is not so easy, even with our family and friends. It does not just come naturally, like blue eyes or black hair. Sometimes we don't feel like behaving lovingly or expressing affection. Sometimes we forget the importance of letting someone know we care. Sarcasm and caustic remarks slip all too easily into our conversation, cutting the stem that connects another to her or his worth.

Some days, we could not care less about what someone has to tell us. Our own agenda hangs so heavily on our minds that we find it very difficult to hear someone else. Those tend to be the days when we learn less.

Loving in the context of professional caregiving has often been viewed as dangerous to the one doing the caring. Many nurses, physicians, and other care providers receive messages urging them not to care too much for fear of burnout. They fear letting go of the familiar model of detached objectivity. They worry about becoming overinvolved and losing their therapeutic perspective.[2]

Carol Leppanen Montgomery, an assistant professor of nursing at the University of Colorado, discovered in her research into the nature of caring from a caregiver's perspective, an overriding theme of spiritual transcendence. Nurses who maintained a level of excellence and work satisfaction described their caring experience as being influenced by a relationship with a force greater than self.

The spiritual dimension of caring includes three properties. The first is the nature of the connection, the unique spiritual nature of the relationship that distinguishes it from what we commonly refer to as overinvolvement, rescuing, or codependency. The second property, the source of energy, explains how spiritual transcendence serves as an important resource for caregiver self-renewal and motivation. It associates caring with profound fulfillment and growth rather than burnout. The third property of spiritual caring is that the effect on the caregiver is one of personal fulfillment rather than emotional depletion.

Love, at this level, becomes a simple act of connection rather than an achievement-oriented act of curing disease or eliminating problems. When we offer care at the level of spirit, we express an understanding of life as fundamentally interconnected, of a common humanity in relationship with one another. This kind of caring underscores many things about love's connection to health and human development. For example, a potent factor in the development of children is the quality of love they receive. The same could be said about the protection of health or the recovery from illness. Love breeds love and other rich possibilities. Intimacy breaks down the experience of being separate. Violence engenders violence. Indifference fosters indifference. Love invites expansion, growth, and health. Intimacy builds supportive relationships. Violence damages life, leaving it small and sickly. Indifference spawns cynicism, apathy, and dryness. Knowing this, how could we intentionally choose anything except love?

Compassion comes from the same cloth as love. A frequently misunderstood healing asset, compassion means far more than expressing pity and pitiful feelings. Pity sometimes regards its object as not only suffering but also as weak and inferior. Compassion does not. It considers nothing and nobody weak or inferior. Compassion works from strength, born of awareness that we humans share our weaknesses. Compassion lifts up and acts mercifully. There is justice-making in compassion.

Like love, compassion cannot be contained in feelings or sentiment. For example, biblical compassion, both in the Hebrew scriptures and in the New Testament, emphasizes action and doing "works of mercy." Jesus' teaching on compassion derives much of its insight from the Jewish spirituality in which he was born and raised. The feeling of compassion in Jesus always gave rise to an outward act of mercy. He healed, he cleansed, and he fed. Compassion as a feeling separated from action would have been inconceivable to Jesus. Like love, compassion is a vocation, a call to serve another. Compassion could be called the world's richest energy source, yet it remains astonishingly underdeveloped.

So what is going on—or, maybe more to the point, what is not going on—in our health care world? How do we tap the wealth of healing energy found in love and compassion? How do we begin to look at our own spirituality and its relationship to our own health and the health of those we care for?

I think we begin when we realize that genuine spirituality constitutes much more than an institutional religious notion. No matter what religious or cultural tradition shapes our beliefs, we cannot legitimately separate the sacred from the secular. How we live out each day is who we are. Our social, political, and economic priorities are the staging ground for crucial spiritual issues of power and love, generosity and selfishness, violence and compassion. Consequently, we need to look at those priorities when we wish to know what is going on with concepts like love and compassion.

I think we also begin to consider spirituality's links with health when we accept the fact that each of our lives matters. How we choose to live our life matters. We have been loved into life by a creator who invites us to share that love with the world in which we live. Whether we are teachers, homemakers, grandparents, or physicians, who we are and what we contribute to this fabric that we call creation has much more impact on others than most of us are willing to believe. Our acts of mercy truly do make a difference. We need to say, simply, "I choose to act in a just and compassionate manner because I am loved and love acts through me. I will help someone for no other reason than that she or he needs help."

COMPASSION AS THE GROUND FOR HEALING

We all possess healing skills that we can share, at any given moment, with others and ourselves. These skills are simple, but powerful: a quiet presence, a capacity to listen, and a posture of hospitality. In addition:

• Caring, considered as pulling from abundance rather than as ego centered, implies the existence of some greater force.

• A healing role includes the recognition that social support, prayer, ritual, and other manifestations of spirituality are significant dimensions in the dynamics of faith and healing. To mobilize these resources on a patient's behalf is both essential and filled with potential.

• We must recognize the value of having one's questions about meaning and hope taken seriously by a caring community or person.

• Giving voice to despair and grief opens both the sufferer and the healer to unanticipated strength with which to endure or transcend crisis. It can give strength to those who live with chronic conditions and those who treat them.

• Making connections with friends, family, and other caregivers fosters the goal of health for health care professionals, for patients, and for families and other day-to-day caregivers.

"Do we create or destroy?" asks Dag Hammarskjöld in his classic *Markings*. Living out compassion is an act of creation. If words like "love" and "compassion" have suffered from excess or misunderstanding, it might be because we have forgotten where they really belong. This whole experience that we call life is really a single lesson, which lies at the heart of health. That lesson begins with a question, "How do we care for ourselves and each other?"

GRATITUDE   *Gratitude acknowledges thankfulness; a feeling of gracious appreciation for favors or benefits received from the hands of another; to take this attitude is to be beholden and grateful for life as a whole rather than only for specific things. A grateful person is one who accepts life in its entirety as fundamentally good and meaningful; gratitude implies sincerity and gladness of spirit. To assume a stance of gratitude is to discover wholeness.*

CHAPTER 29

A Reason to Hope

◦✥◦

I said to the night
That stood at the gate of the new year,
"Give me a light
that I might tread safely
into the dark and unknown."
And a voice said in reply,
"Put your hand into the hand of the one who made you,
and your reward will be
blessed with more light
far safer
than the unknown."

—Author unknown

WHEN I ASKED HIM the meaning of hope, a wise friend told me, "Most people tend to associate hope with optimism. I find it more helpful to define the optimist as someone who says everything is going to be fine. The pessimist says everything will be awful. The hopeful person says, 'However things shall be, God can and will bring forth life.'"

This must be true, for there are many situations in which we have no reason for optimism, but every reason for hope.

One of those occasions took place in the month of January. The young parents in the emergency room watched without words as a team of physicians, pharmacists, respiratory therapists, nurses, and more labored over their baby boy. Hoping against hope, the man and woman gripped each other's hands and prayed together for a miracle that would revive their son.

Born just a few weeks earlier, Stephen had been diagnosed with hemophilia, though, by all accounts, he was doing very well. Surprised at their good fortune of an unplanned pregnancy, both Stephen's parents and his older siblings were thrilled at the baby boy's arrival. The instant he emerged from his mother's womb, he became the cooing center of his family's adoration. His ecstatic parents clucked attentively over his every move, keeping a watchful eye on all aspects of his care.

This morning, however, something had gone terribly wrong. Somewhere between a family rejoicing at breakfast over their exquisite son and the father's drive home from a visit with relatives, Stephen died. He produced not a sound, not a seizure, not a hint of warning. He simply stopped breathing. More shocking, his father did not discover the catastrophe until he parked the car in the garage and reached into the backseat to lift Stephen from his infant seat. In an instant, the mystery of love that created him and prepared a place for him was about to come to terms with letting him go.

After what seemed an interminable hour, the emergency room physician in charge of resuscitation efforts stopped and looked helplessly into the parents' faces. It was hardly necessary for her to speak, as everyone had known or at least suspected the outcome before the painstaking attempt to revive Stephen even began. The rest of the trauma team backed away from the baby, paralyzed by agony and disbelief. It was sudden infant death syndrome. It was over.

What happened next, however, would transform this devastating loss into a life-altering experience of a very different nature. Stephen's parents, crushed beyond description, turned to the group and thanked each person in the room for her or his valiant effort to save Stephen's life. The couple then thanked each other for the

life they had shared for many years. They thanked their family
physician and the clinic nurses who had provided Stephen's ongoing care. They even thanked the paramedics who raced to their
home and toiled in vain to breathe life back into Stephen.

Finally, though tearful and shaky, Stephen's father gently
wrapped his son in a clean receiving blanket, lifted the baby
upward toward the blinding trauma room lights, thanked God for
sharing Stephen with him and with his family, and then baptized
the lifeless child. It was a gesture of gratitude that brought the
normally bustling emergency department to a speechless standstill.
The tables had turned. A family who had lost more than words
could say had extended a healing hand and heartfelt gratitude to
the professional caregivers.

"There is no tragedy, nor is there any kind of loss, through
which life cannot come forward," said Stephen's father several
weeks later. "Sometimes we simply have no control, and all we
can do is try to go on living our lives with integrity. Stephen's
death was outside of our control, but we trust that life can come
from it. We know grace can be in it."

Several months later, Stephen's physician was to offer the
address at a hospital memorial service held for all the families
whose children had died in the past year. Before an auditorium full
of pensive people, he spoke about mercy and gratitude and how
important a role both played in the practice of medicine. He then
simply thanked the members of the audience. He thanked them for
teaching him about children and for allowing him to care for their
children. He thanked them for sharing their wisdom about loss
with him. Then he told them a story about the death of his father.

What a long and difficult path the two had walked together
through his father's treatment for debilitating heart disease. The
doctor described the gratitude he felt for his father's life and how
the two of them had made a point of expressing their appreciation
for the blessings of a shared life. He talked about compassion and
spoke with simplicity of heart about how it felt to have no cure
to offer. Eventually, he told the story of his father's last hours, the

bathing and gently turning him and changing of his bedclothes.
He described massaging his father's feet and hands, all the tender
care that prevails when clinical practice becomes moot. At the end,
each man said thank you to the other and to the silence. And then
they said good-bye.

After witnessing both of those events, I realized that there are
some things in life we can take into our hands and hold up to
the light or put under a microscope for a clearer understanding.
We can sift through a handful of pebbles or inspect a beautiful
piece of silk. We can perceive the magnificence of a masterful
painting; we can observe the petals of a rose. But there are other
matters that we cannot grasp with our hands or eyes, but only
with our hearts. These extend beyond our reach and our comprehension. They carry us past the conscious world of familiar
scenery and sounds into a silent world of the unknown. Some
would describe these experiences as encounters with mystery,
the revelation of something hidden. In the case of the family
and the physician the mystery originates in their posture of gratitude for all of life—life blessed and life broken. Father to son.
Son to father. Theirs was an unbroken circle of mercy and gratitude, a connection of the heart that begins in life and remains
in death.

Stephen died in the month of January. January receives its
name from Janus, the god of thresholds. Janus is often pictured
with two faces. One face looks backward in memory, and the
other face searches the horizon of the future. Janus is also the
patron of doorways. The month that bears his name marks
the season of endings and beginnings, as in the beginning of a
new year. It is the time of inventories. January is the month of
resuming old routines after the holidays and starting new ones
that sustain us through the rest of the winter.

The ability to assume a posture of gratitude does not make
crossing the January threshold and beginning anew any less dif-

ficult or painful. Beginnings and endings never come easily. Adjusting life plans and reshaping lost dreams takes tremendous courage. To adapt their vision and their direction is a challenge that stands before Stephen's family, before their physician, and before most of us much of the time. These are the things that sometimes make us wonder if we should stretch out our hand to welcome another day, or turn over and pull the blanket over our head. Shall we hide from life, or shall we embrace it? Can *we* find a reason to hope?

January is an invitation to each of us to stand at the threshold of life. It's a season for looking over who we are and asking ourselves where we're going. Do we like what we see? Are we growing and taking risks? Do we know how to take care of ourselves and live well? Can we follow our hearts into the cold and recognize signs of new life amid all the trials and blessings we face? Do we want to be well?

Most of us experience growth and understanding of our journeys in fleeting glimpses rather than in dramatic turning points. Truth unfolds slowly more often than it appears in great flashes of light. Its pattern remains hidden beneath the routine events of the day. Even if hope tells us our lives have a direction and a destiny, it's only in gifted moments that we gain enough perspective to see this mosaic of meaning.

An ancient Orphic hymn proclaims that the night is the birth of all things. January takes us out into the bitter cold; yet, for Stephen's parents and for his doctor, the darkness of January was not a night of despair, but a night of watching for the light of January. They came to realize that in life as in death, we are truly linked together by a most fragile thread. Creation and compassion give birth to this delicate link. Gratitude and mercy sustain it.

We have known for a half-century that all else being equal, sick people plummet when hopelessness paralyzes them. Hope is a therapeutic agent every bit as essential as antibodies.

Janice Post-White, a University of Minnesota researcher and professor of oncology nursing, says that hope constitutes a key spiritual element of healing to which medical professionals should pay careful attention. Hope provides purpose, direction, and a reason for being.

In an effort to unearth the meaning and value of hope, Post-White began by defining hope as "the search for meaning and existential purpose in life in relation to self, others, and a higher being." Next, she and a team of researchers at the University of Minnesota Cancer Center interviewed thirty-two cancer patients. What they discovered was that, besides finding meaning through formal religion or spirituality, cancer patients also identified five themes or assets related to their capacity to hope:

Inner resources such as character, positive attitudes, self-determination, self-worth, optimism, a strong will, coping processes, humor, and motivation.

Affirming relationships with family, friends, health care professionals, and pets; feeling needed, valued, and cared for; enjoyment in relationships; the experience of others being present and available.

Present living, which involves living in the moment; a sense of normalcy; getting through; keeping busy; physical independence; quality of life.

Anticipating survival or expecting positive results from treatment and/or cure; receiving positive information; considering the future; waiting for events; finding a purpose in living.[1]

Post-White further learned that health care professionals can encourage hope in cancer patients by giving information in a positive manner, demonstrating caring behavior, and simply being available and present. Conversely, health care professionals take away a patient's hope when they assume a disrespectful, cold, or blunt manner or give discouraging medical information without also giving patients something to hold on to. Overall, patients in the study revealed that tending to spiritual and physical needs is important to hope and to the quality of life of cancer survivors.

Appendix

If listening lies at the heart of health, asking the right questions and using language that everyone can understand help to shape people's responses to illness. The following definitions, inventories, and questions offer some discussion opportunities for patients and doctors.

HELPFUL LANGUAGE

Cure   To find a remedy or solution that engenders complete recovery or correction of disease; restoration of health; an event brought about through medical manipulation having to do with nonspiritual aspects of one's disease or illness.

Healing   An internal process that draws on one's emotional, physical, and spiritual resources; a process of becoming freed to move beyond brokenness. Healing may not change the medical outcome, but it increases a person's sense of well-being by fostering feelings of safety, confidence, wholeness, and hope.

Health   Absence of significant disease or excessive conflict, pain, and anxiety; an ability to function effectively and in a reasonably good mood; some sense of self-discipline and a capacity to love and feel connected to others. Whether someone is healthy is a value judgment involving input from both patient and physician.

Illness The partial or complete absence of the valuable asset called health; the presence of disease and, with it, a threat to a person's feelings of connection and meaning.

Hope Relates to expectancy, which is distinctly different from expectations; a stance of the heart that is open to whatever life might bring, having no agenda but anticipating future good.

Meaning The background against which humankind asks spiritual questions such as "Who am I? From where have I come? Where am I going? What is the purpose and value of my life?" With regard to illness, meaning is at least as important as diagnosis.

Creation In relation to illness, means creating order out of chaos; pointing to how a person can preserve or reintroduce structure and shape to life; establishing routines, familiar patterns, and life-sustaining organization.

Courage A quality that allows one to move forward in the face of fear and ambiguity; to encourage others is to share courage, to nurture, and to create an environment in which another can move toward hope; it sets the stage for a fruitful outcome.

A SPIRITUAL INVENTORY FOR A HEALING MODEL

A growing body of medical literature suggests that spirituality is of interest and benefit to both patients and health practitioners. There have been no helpful tools with which to measure spirituality, though asking questions such as the following can contribute valuable information to an individual's health history. The questions also help patients address concerns about their health condition before those worries grow to unmanageable proportions.

What is going on in your life, especially with your family, other people important to you, and your work?

How do you feel about the things taking place in your life?

What keeps you awake at night or troubles you the most?

How do you cope with the things that trouble you the most?

Who is your primary source of emotional support in difficult times?

Do you fully understand your current health situation?

How do you feel about it?

Why do you think you have become ill at this time?

What is most difficult for you about being sick?

BREAKING BAD NEWS

Parents of 189 children enrolled in 15 developmental day care centers completed questionnaires that surveyed the experience of receiving bad news from their physicians. The study elicited preferences for physician behavior in a hypothetical situation. The strongest preferences included:

Ninety-seven percent preferred that physicians show a caring attitude

Ninety-five percent wished that parents be allowed to talk

Ninety-five percent desired that parents be allowed to show their own feelings

Ninety percent wanted physicians to share information

Eighty-nine percent wished for physicians to be highly confident

Eighty-seven percent desired parent-to-parent referral

Nineteen percent actually received a referral to another parent[1]

The study showed a difference between what parents experienced and what they desired in physicians who communicate bad news. According to these parents, they preferred that the physician be in control of such an interaction and be highly confident, but also demonstrate caring and allow parents to talk and share their feelings.

Parents Want Information

The physician who breaks bad news to families is an important one. This is the person who introduces a family to their child's future. If the physician's behavior inspires trust and cooperation, the family tends to approach the future more readily. If the physician's behavior is difficult, the parents may have difficulty accepting their child's health condition, complying with treatment, and remaining hopeful. A few helpful guidelines for physicians and friends:

> Avoid intellectualizing.
> Let pain be pain.
> Realize that there is no rational answer to human suffering.
> Be prepared to listen and to admit that you have no answers.
> Accept that you can't fix everything, but know that you always have something to offer your patients.
> Know that you are human and that is enough.

A Physician's Spiritual Self-Assessment

God

> Do you feel there is a God or a power greater than yourself?
> If so, describe that greater power (e.g., is it unknowable, distant, vulnerable, present, omnipotent, angry?).
> Does this God have an active role in the current human condition? Does this God care?

Your Choice to Become a Physician

> Who were your role models when you were young?
> Who or what influenced your choice to become a physician? What did you think doctors could do?

As you grew up, did you or your family identify with a
particular religious tradition or cultural belief system?
Explain.

Describe how your own spirituality or belief system
influences your role as a health care professional.

Have your experiences of religion or other beliefs
influenced your idea of life's meaning or the way you
practice medicine? If so, how?

Health and Illness

How would you describe health?

How would you describe illness?

Describe your personal experience with illness. Did you
feel alone, cared for, neglected?

Who cared for you when you were sick?

What are your current views about death—is it a medical
mistake, a failure, or something else?

Your Role as a Physician-Healer

What kind of relationship do you prefer to have with a
patient/family?

What do you give your patients? How do they benefit
most from having you as their physician? How do they
benefit least?

Aside from taking a health history, what kinds of questions
are you apt to ask patients? What kinds of questions are
you apt to ask their family?

How do you suppose knowing a patient's spiritual issues—
conflicts, fears, anxieties, and so on—could help you
diagnose and care for them?

The Art of the Healer

If you were an outside observer, how would you describe
yourself as a physician?

What was the last thing you did for a patient—other than provide prescription drugs or some kind of clinical intervention—that made him or her feel good?

How did it make you feel?

When was the last occasion on which you spent much time with a patient (or the family of a patient) whom you viewed as already a medical failure? What kind of experience was that for you?

Self-Care

As a caregiver, what do you think others expect of you? What do you expect of yourself?

What is the most important thing you have learned in life? In your profession?

What are your own problems, issues, or conflicts with peers, family, and others?

What gets you up in the morning? What do you live for and look forward to?

Do you think that reflecting on and discussing (with another person) your own spiritual concerns, conflicts, and fears would be beneficial to you as a caregiver? How?

If you were to discuss these issues with someone, whom would you choose as the listener—a colleague, mate, minister, other?

Do you feel you have an adequate support system? Do you have a space in which you can be vulnerable and free from judgment? Have you had adequate spiritual support throughout your medical training?

If you tried to describe your life as a journey, in what stage of the process would you say you found yourself today? Where would you like to be? How do you plan to get there?

Source Notes

Chapter 7: To Some, Health Is a Value Judgment

1. Hippocrates, *Human Medicine,* Toronto Western Hospital, Toronto, Canada, 1998, p. 85.

Chapter 8: Doctors Need to Remember Their Roles as Healers

1. Larry Dossey, M.D., *Common Boundary,* vol. 15, no. 3, March/April 1997, p. 41.
2. *Ibid,* p. 42.
3. Paul Tournier, M.D., *A Listening Ear,* Augsburg Fortress Publishing House, Minneapolis, MN, 1980, p. 28.

Chapter 14: Nourishing the Body Can Heal the Soul

1. Deborah Kesten, *Feeding the Body, Nourishing the Soul,* Conari Press, Berkeley, Cal., 1997, pp. 55–120.

Chapter 16: The Courage to Cope with Chronic Illness

1. Catherine Hoffman, Dorothy Rice, and Hai-Yen Sung, "Persons with Chronic Conditions: Their Prevalence and Costs," *Journal of the American Medical Association,* vol. 276, no. 18, November 13, 1996, pp. 1473–1479.

Chapter 17: Looking for Meaning

1. Parker J. Palmer, *The Company of Strangers: Christians and the Renewal of American Public Life,* Crossroad, New York, NY, 1981, p. 44.

Chapter 23: The Role of Spiritual Development in Health

1. Thomas C. Ogden, *Agenda for Theology: Recovering Christian Roots,* Harper & Row, New York, 1979, pp. 36–38.
2. Edward P. Wimberly, "Spirituality and Health: Caring in a Postmodern Age," *The Caregiver Journal,* vol. 12, no. 4, 1996.

Chapter 24: The Power of Story

1. Robert Coles, *The Call of Stories,* Houghton Mifflin, Boston, 1990, pp. 7–10.

Chapter 25: Cultivating the Art of Being

1. Gunilla Norris, *Sharing Silence,* Crown Publishers, Inc., 1992, p. 19.
2. H. G. Koenig, L. B. Bearon, and R. Dayringer, "Physicians' Perspectives on the Role of Religion in the Physician-Older Patient Relationship," *Family Practice,* vol. 28, 1989, pp. 441–448.

Chapter 28: The Heart of Health

1. Dean Ornish, M.D., "All You Need Is Love," *New Age: The Journal for Holistic Living,* 1998–99, p. 18.
2. Carol Leppanen Montgomery, RN, Ph.D., "The Care Giving Relationship: Paradoxical and Transcendent Aspects," *Alternative Therapies,* vol. 2, no. 2, March 1996, pp. 52–57.

Chapter 29: A Reason to Hope

1. Janice Post-White, RN, Ph.D., "Hope, Spirituality, Sense of Coherence, and Quality of Life in Patients with Cancer," *Oncology Nursing Forum,* vol. 23, no. 10, Nov.–Dec. 1996, pp. 1571–1579.

Appendix

1. Michael Sharp, Ronald Strauss, and Sharon Claire Lorch, "Communicating Medical Bad News: Parents' Experiences and Preferences," *The Journal of Pediatrics,* vol. 121, no. 4, October 1992, pp. 539–546.